CW01019769

20/05

YOU
FAT LOSS
JOURNEY STARTS HERE

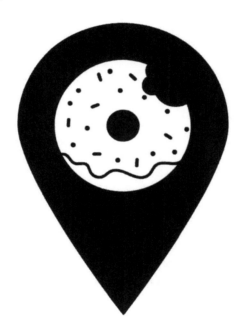

Ditch the Diets
Gain More Confidence
Be Forever in Control

LEONARDO ALVES

ISBN: 978-989-35913-0-7 (Hardcover)
ISBN: 978-989-35913-1-4 (Paperback)
ISBN: 978-989-35913-2-1 (Kindle Ebook)

Table of Contents

Chapter 1:
Understanding Fat Loss

Imagine we're grabbing a relaxed coffee together—a dash of milk and no sugar for me—and I mention something we see everywhere these days: weight loss.

You've seen it, right? Plastered on magazine covers, flooding your digital platforms, and shaping how you see yourself. It's like everyone around you has turned into a weight loss guru overnight, each with their own secret method for shedding pounds.

I know it's ironic to bring up weight loss when it's already everywhere, but here's why we need to talk about it: it's time for a straight-up, no-nonsense chat.

As a personal trainer and 1-2-1 online fitness coach with thousands of interactions on the gym floor and online, I see firsthand that many people are left confused, which is precisely why we're here. These mixed messages make it tricky to figure out what really works.

So, despite the 1,001 theories floating around, the basics of how fat loss happens are pretty simple. At its core, it's about energy—what we consume and burn. But the world's obsession with quick fixes, 'revolutionary' methods, and the eagerness to make a quick buck has often drowned out this truth.

However, just because it's straightforward physiologically, it doesn't mean every other aspect is easy. The more significant challenges can lie mentally, habitually, and even socially.

Before continuing our chat, here's something important: if you don't want to focus on fat loss, that's perfectly fine. It's your choice. The world of fitness and health is enormous, with countless other aims you might be interested in, and we'll go into those later.

But if you're here for the fat loss journey, I'm here to support you.

So, before we dive into the details, let's make a promise: we'll keep it real, stick to the facts, and support each other every step of the way.

Are you in?

You Can't Screw This Up

Picture this: I'm in South London, in my early 20s, just chilling, when I decide to grab some takeaway fried chicken from a local shop. Sounds pretty harmless, right? Well, sometimes after something like that, I'd be beating myself up, thinking I need to do extra at the gym or with my nutrition to make up for it. But this one time, I didn't. I just kept on with my usual routine.

Surprisingly, I continued to see strength gains and hit a new low on the scale and measurements days later.

Had I convinced myself that I had 'screwed everything up' and quit, I would have missed seeing the progress that was just around the corner.

So, before we dive deeper into all the nitty-gritty of fitness, I share that brief story so that I can tell you straight up: *you cannot screw up your fitness journey.*

Seriously.

You cannot screw it up.

You might be thinking, 'That's not true, Leo. Give me 20 minutes, and I can mess up my fitness journey with not only fried chicken, but a large pizza, a box of doughnuts, and a bag of cookies with extra chocolate chips.'

Here's the reality: even if you did indulge in all that, you haven't "ruined" anything.

Yes, devouring a large pepperoni pizza, half a dozen glazed doughnuts, and a bag of cookies at once isn't the best idea. Plus, if it's a frequent occurrence, it's worth exploring why.

But this notion of 'screwing up' is precisely what could be holding you back.

Fitness isn't a switch you flick on and off. It's a lifelong journey. Embracing it as an ongoing part of your life makes the process much more manageable and less intimidating. This shift in perspective is precisely why many of my 1-2-1 online fitness members have stayed consistent with their health and fitness for years. It helps you recognise that you're always just one decision, meal, or workout away from a positive step forward.

With this mindset in place, let's lightly touch on a few other essential topics before we dive deeper into everything else. Starting with skewed and unrealistic expectations.

Skewed and Unrealistic Expectations

Let me tell you about Melissa, an East Londoner, passionate dog lover, and one of my 1-2-1 online fitness members. A few months into us working together, she expressed frustration during a call. She felt she wasn't progressing enough and thought she should do more. I simply replied, 'You realise that out of all my 1-2-1 online fitness members, you're perhaps crushing it the most right now?' (She seriously was doing a fantastic job.)

That moment of recognition changed everything for her. Over two years later, she's still making incredible strides.

Why do I bring this up?

Well, Melissa's initial frustration is something many of us feel on our fitness journeys, especially when unrealistic expectations bog us down. After all, your fitness motivation is heavily influenced by what you think is realistically achievable.

Consider this analogy from football: scoring a hat-trick (3 goals in one game) is terrific. But you wouldn't appreciate the achievement if you didn't know much about football and thought "just 3 goals" was average or a poor showing. Similarly, if you embark on your fitness journey with skewed expectations, it's easy to undervalue your progress. So, understanding and setting realistic goals is vital for maintaining a positive outlook and recognising your achievements.

The most common example of this is a statement like 'Leo, I've only lost 3kg in the past 3 months,' usually said with a sense of frustration.

But let's zoom into this type of statement for a moment.

4

'Only' 3kg, according to who? What standard are you measuring against? Losing 3kg is still a terrific achievement. It's especially something to shout home about in a world where obesity rates are rising. If you've struggled with fat loss for years, any progress is a victory worth celebrating. Every step forward counts—the same way every piece placed in a puzzle is progress towards completing the picture.

Moreover, consider the broader context of your journey.

Perhaps this time, you made progress without sacrificing your social life or restricting yourself from your favourite foods. It may be the first time you've adopted a healthier, more balanced approach to exercise.

It's crucial to recognise and appreciate your progress rather than downplaying it. You wouldn't dismiss a friend's achievements, so be kind to yourself. Each step forward, no matter how small it seems, is a step in the right direction.

The Truth About Fitness and Fat Loss

Despite what some eager-to-profit gurus or the teenager with endless time for workouts and meal prep might claim, fat loss can be challenging.

There will be days when quitting seems easier than continuing, when skipping the gym is tempting, and moments when it feels like you're the only one not seeing results. If you've tried losing weight before, you know this feeling well.

It's also easy to find reasons to delay progress. Before working together, my 1-2-1 online fitness member Matt used to make excuses to put off his fitness goals, especially after returning from vacation. He'd tell himself he'd start again later, and those "breaks" often lasted months. But after returning from a trip to India, something clicked. He realised he could stay committed throughout the year, and now, no matter what, he crushes it.

This brings us to an important lesson about breaking limits.

It reminds me of Roger Bannister's story. Before 1954, it was widely believed that no one could run a mile in under 4 minutes—it just wasn't humanly possible, or so everyone thought. Then Bannister ran a mile in 3 minutes 59.4 seconds, proving the limits people had accepted weren't real. Since then, countless runners have broken that record, even at the collegiate level.

Both Matt's experience and Bannister's feat teach us a vital lesson: sometimes, the biggest obstacle isn't the physical challenge—it's the belief that we can't succeed. Once you recognise that success is possible, those barriers—whether it's procrastination or a 4-minute mile—start to fall.

Let's move on to the next section, where we'll distinguish a key difference.

Fat Loss v Weight Loss

While the terms "fat loss" and "weight loss" are often used interchangeably— admittedly, I sometimes do this too—it's essential to understand the difference between the 2 in the context of our chat. Knowing this difference will significantly increase your understanding of everything we're about to discuss.

Weight loss can result from various factors, such as reductions in body fat and muscle mass, trips to the toilet, hydration levels, sodium intake, cutting off one's leg, or even illnesses–I remember getting food poisoning at work one time and losing almost 2 kg in 24 hours (don't ask). These are all examples that can lead to significant fluctuations in the scale.

On the other hand, fat loss is solely a reduction in body fat. Unlike the daily fluctuations seen in body weight, changes in body fat occur more slowly, either subtly increasing, decreasing, or stabilising over time.

Achieving weight loss is generally more straightforward than specifically targeting body fat. For instance, extreme calorie restriction without considering nutrients or a specific plan behind your workouts can lead to weight loss. However, this type of approach is unhealthy in the long run. It will often cause you to feel worse due to decreased valuable muscle mass, a lack of calories and nutritious food to fuel your daily life.

Therefore, our chat focuses on fat loss—the process of reducing body fat healthily and in a way that'll stick. This involves adopting dietary habits that are right for you and maintaining or building muscle mass, which is crucial for a strong, healthy body.

Next up: the term "diet."

The Term "Diet"

Throughout our chat, you'll notice that I sometimes use the term "diet." I want to be clear that, unless I specify otherwise, I'm not talking about extreme eating plans where you have to give up all the foods you love, only drink shakes, or try a useless detox that only leaves you on the toilet for a few days.

What I mean by "diet" is simply the food and drink you regularly have.

I say this because it's crucial to understand that diets aren't inherently "bad"—which is a tiring narrative consistently circulating.

Some people have a specific diet to help them gain weight.

Some have a specific diet due to religious reasons.

Others have a specific diet because of allergies or intolerances, such as myself, who avoids garlic and onion. (My wife huffs at having to exclude these whenever she decides to cook.)

Diets themselves aren't inherently negative.

How you approach your diet, known as how you eat, makes it good or bad.

Let's break it down a bit more.

Upon looking up the definition, the word "diet" has 2 main meanings:

- One is "A special course of food to which a person restricts themselves, either to lose weight or for medical reasons."
- But I'm mainly using it in the second sense: "The kinds of food that a person, animal, or community habitually eats."

With this understanding, we can now expand on the most critical point for fat loss: calories.

The Importance of Calories and the Calorie Deficit

The most important factor for fat loss is a calorie deficit. Without a calorie deficit, shedding fat isn't possible. Now, you might be curious about what exactly a calorie deficit is. Simply put, it means that the calories you consume from foods and drinks are less than your body burns daily. By burns, I'm talking about everything your body does—digesting foods, fidgeting, or even laughing at memes all contributing.

Think of calories as your body's fuel for all its activities.

If the calories you eat and drink match what you burn, you're at calorie maintenance. This means your body will stay at its current weight, typically within a one or two-kilogram range (2.2-4.4 lbs).

However, if you eat and drink more calories than your body needs, the excess is stored as fat. This is known as a calorie surplus and is your body's way of saving energy for later.

Let's dive in further with an example.

Suppose your body needs between 1,900 and 2,100 calories daily to maintain weight. Eating and drinking less than this range puts you in a calorie deficit, while eating more results in a calorie surplus.

For instance:

- Consuming 1,550 calories a day means you're in a calorie deficit.
- Having 1,950 calories a day is maintaining your calorie balance.
- Taking in 2,600 calories a day would lead to a calorie surplus.

Now that we've established this, let's look at how other popular "weight loss diets" take the concept of a calorie deficit but give it a fancy name and rules to entice the consumer:

- Keto: Eliminates an entire food group.
- Intermittent Fasting: Cuts out an entire meal.
- Carnivore: Restricts you to only meat/eggs.
- Vegan: Removes all animal-based foods.
- 5:2: Greatly limits eating on 2 days of the week.
- Paleo: Excludes foods not consumed by our ancient ancestors.

- **Low-Fat Diet:** Minimises intake of the most calorie-dense macronutrient.
- The "avoid any food that's blue, contains more than 3 syllables in its name, or begins with the letter C and isn't a protein source, fruit, or vegetable" diet: This one's made up, but you get the point.

I know some of these nutrition approaches have purposes beyond fat loss, such as veganism for ethical reasons or keto for what it was initially intended for, which was epilepsy. However, I'm explicitly discussing people who start those nutrition approaches to lose fat—and it's in this context the Dunning-Kruger effect can often manifest.

This psychological phenomenon occurs when people with limited knowledge or expertise in a particular area overestimate their abilities or expertise. Essentially, they don't know enough to realise how little they know, leading them to proclaim the "extraordinary effectiveness" of these trendy diets for fat loss without fully understanding their broader implications or suitability for others. However, it's not the diet that's magic—it's that by applying these arbitrary rules, you potentially increase your chances of consuming fewer calories overall.

Now, this isn't to say you should or shouldn't eat in a specific way or a dick-measuring contest about who has the best diet, because I'm all for the message that if you've found a nutrition approach that works for you, is healthy, and helps you make progress, then go for it. I'm just highlighting that there's nothing magical about these approaches for fat loss beyond the calorie deficit they'll potentially put you in.

What I will say, though, is that when it comes to fat loss specifically, if your diet has a name, then chances are, it's not a good idea.

Anyway, understanding calories in foods can also help you see that no single food item will automatically cause weight gain. It's not about just one chocolate bar, a slice of bread, a bowl of cereal, a spoonful of olive oil, or a glass of fruit juice. For example, my 1-2-1 online fitness member, cat lover and audiobook enjoyer, Anca, lost 10kg of body fat and reached her best shape ever while enjoying a chocolate bar most days. What matters for sustainable fat loss is whether you consistently consume slightly fewer calories than you burn over time.

Now, bear with me—this isn't to say that all foods have the same nutritional value either—far from it.

Sure, a calorie's a calorie. After all, it's a unit of measurement. In the same way, a mile is a mile, regardless of whether it's in the jungle or the desert. But the source of that calorie can and will make all the difference in how we feel, function, and even look. Two foods might have the same calories but can play entirely different roles in your body. For example, a 100-calorie sugary treat and a 100-calorie hearty salad have 100 calories but are worlds apart nutritionally.

Your nutrition should consist mainly of single-ingredient, minimally processed, high-protein, and high-fibre foods. That's not to say you shouldn't hesitate to include some more "fun" foods, too—I find prioritising the former while sprinkling in the latter gives me and my 1-2-1 online fitness members a lovely middle ground.

To wrap up this calorie talk, I understand that a calorie deficit might seem straightforward—use more calories than you consume, and you'll lose fat. However, the reality of fat loss, fitness, and life aren't always so simple. Various factors influence this equation, including the types of foods you eat, how your metabolism functions, your level of physical activity, and more. We'll speak about all of these—hence the reason for this whole coffee shop chat.

This brings us to our next topic, nutrition essentials for fat loss.

Chapter 2:
Nutrition Essentials for Fat Loss

While we sit at this coffee shop and wait for our drinks to finish being prepared, it's a great time to touch on the fact that the importance of nutrition isn't a new understanding. It dates back to 460 B.C. (imagine what the world must've been like then) with Hippocrates, a renowned Greek physician, who famously said, *"Let food be your medicine and medicine be your food."* His wisdom still echoes today, highlighting the power of what you eat and drink.

Now, you've probably encountered countless bits of nutrition advice. From strict dietary rules to numerous weight loss tips, there's no shortage of everything ranging from excellent to awful information. In addition, navigating the world of nutrition is becoming increasingly overwhelming. When you enter the cereal aisle at your local grocery store, consider the countless choices, ranging from "kid-friendly" sugary options to health-focused cereals, budget brands, and an array of granolas and mueslis.

Many food categories present a similar array of choices.

In this upcoming part of our chat, coffee in hand, let's share a laugh over some of the outrageous diet myths, separating everything that's fact from hype.

Macronutrients and Micronutrients Explained:

Two of the most fundamental aspects of nutrition are macronutrients and micronutrients.

If you know what they are, great!

If you're raising an eyebrow, you're good too—because by the end of this part of the conversation, you'll be able to educate the next person on the must-knows.

Here's a brief introduction to each.

Macronutrients: The Big Players

- **Proteins:** Think of these as the building blocks. Protein ensures everything's strong and working—from your muscles to hunger levels to the tiniest hair strands. Meats and seafood are excellent sources. I'll speak about protein in more depth shortly, but for now, know that protein has 4 calories per gram.

- **Carbohydrates:** Carbs often get blamed for fat gain, although they don't inherently make you fat. If you don't believe me, all you have to do is look at Japan, which has one of the lowest obesity rates and highest life expectancies in the world, and they often eat white rice. Carbs are our primary source of energy. Think of them like the fuel you put in your car. They'll get you through those demanding martial arts, marathons or gym sessions. They come in 2 forms: simple (sugars) and complex (fibres and starches). Foods like bread, rice, potatoes and fruits are rich in carbohydrates. Like protein, these also contain 4 calories per gram.

- **Fats:** Many people also think that fat makes you fat—but the fat found in food isn't the same as body fat. So, before you grimace, know this—healthy fats are your friends (when consumed in moderation). They protect your organs, maintain the health of your cell walls, and some vitamins even need fat to be absorbed properly. Now, where do you find good fats? Avocados, olive oil, nuts, and fatty fish are excellent choices. Fats have 9 calories per gram, making them the most calorie-dense food group—meaning it's easy for daily calorie intake to rack up with these if you aren't mindful.

Now that you understand the basics of what you eat, let's explore how you keep everything functioning smoothly with micronutrients.

Micronutrients: The Sprinkles on Our Dietary Doughnut

When I first decided to go all-in on my health and fitness journey, I knew fruits and vegetables were excellent. However, I was so focused on meticulously hitting my daily calorie, protein, carb, and fat targets that I didn't consider my vitamin and mineral intake. This is one of the pitfalls of an IIFYM (If It Fits Your Macros) approach, where the emphasis on hitting daily calorie goals can sometimes lead you to neglect the quality of food you eat. While my diet did include fruits and vegetables, they weren't a focus, and I wasn't eating them as much as I should've.

Thankfully, as time went on, I opened my eyes, acknowledged their importance, and started to include these frequently—and luckily, that phase of neglect was only brief, so I didn't suffer from any poor health consequences.

I guarantee I would have if I'd persisted for long enough.

So, while macronutrients are important, micronutrients such as vitamins and minerals play massive roles in keeping us healthy.

Vitamins A, the Bs, C, D, and E are examples of vitamins. Minerals are potassium, calcium, magnesium, iron, and zinc. In the same way, every part of a machine is vital for it to work; vitamins and minerals are essential for your body to function optimally. They're involved in various processes, from wound healing to regulating hormones, maintaining a steady heartbeat, and strengthening your bones. Vitamins and minerals ensure you function at your best.

To ensure you get a wide range of these vitamins and minerals, you must eat a balanced diet, including, but not limited to, vegetables, legumes, fruits, fibre, protein sources, and healthy fats.

The Importance of Protein: More Than Just Muscles

Now that we've completed the brief introductions, let's discuss protein more deeply—your body's building blocks.

The importance of protein has been recognised for ages, and a fascinating example of this can be seen from World War II. During this time, the science of nutrition was gaining momentum, and the U.S. government emphasised the necessity of "protective foods" to maintain the health of civilians and military personnel. This suggestion was implemented through concern, as many of the draftees in the USA were rejected due to being deemed malnourished and unfit to serve.

The protective foods included protein-rich items such as milk, eggs, fish, and even organ meats, further proving their critical role in a nutritious diet. There was also a wartime propaganda campaign suggesting that by consuming less of these essential foods, Americans could indirectly be aiding the enemy—Hitler. This campaign highlighted the significance of these foods in maintaining health during challenging times.

This isn't me saying that protein is just meat or seafood. Plant-based options like beans, lentils, and tofu also contain it. So, getting enough protein is doable and delicious.

Switching gears, it's a common misconception that protein's benefits are only for those who work out or want to build muscle. However, what if I told you that protein isn't just helpful if you're looking to bulk up at the gym? Protein is essential for everyone, every day, whether bench pressing or hitting 'snooze' on your old-school alarm clock. It plays a massive role in repairing tissues, helping hormones, and supporting overall health.

You may also be wondering why protein is vital for fat loss specifically.

That's because aside from all the benefits we've already mentioned, it's the macronutrient that will keep you fullest for the longest. While on this fat loss journey and aiming to maintain a calorie deficit, think of protein as your best mate coming in clutch and keeping those hunger pangs at bay. It'll also help ensure that you maintain or build valuable muscle because too little protein can result in muscle loss—which you don't want.

Here are 2 simple ways to figure out your protein goal:

- Aim for about 0.7 to 1 gram per pound of body weight, so if you weigh 180lbs, you could aim for a minimum of 126 grams of protein.
- If you have a lot of body fat to lose, aim for 0.7 to 1 gram per pound of your *goal body weight* instead.

It's also a good idea to aim for a protein "minimum" rather than feeling like you have to hit 126 grams on the dot—if you get more, that's fine, too!

Remember that many people struggle with protein intake once they start tracking and being conscious of it for the first time—this is normal. You need to go through a phase of not totally knowing what you're doing before you become efficient and better—whether it's playing the piano, trying a new video game or eating more daily protein.

So, with that said, if you're looking to increase your protein effortlessly, then a few suggestions to consider are:

- Double your current protein portion sizes.
- Front-load your protein intake at breakfast by aiming for at least 30g. This will help prevent you from feeling like you're always playing catch-up throughout the day.
- Have go-to readily available protein sources within reach.
- Consider protein supplements for convenience—a protein bar or protein powder can work great. Although ideally, only opt for these if you're struggling.
- Have a protein source with every meal. Ideally about 25g+.

Alongside protein, fibre is also important—so let's speak about that!

The Importance of Fibre: Your Digestive System's Best Friend

One of my biggest observations is that the fitness industry frequently discusses calories and protein—both important. However, fibre is commonly overlooked, and it's just as crucial.

Fibre is essential for a healthy digestive system, and it's found mainly in complex carbohydrates. It keeps things moving smoothly in your intestines, preventing constipation—and no one likes to feel constipated.

However, fibre's benefits extend beyond just going to the toilet. It plays a crucial role in weight management, as it helps you feel full for longer, which results in you reducing the likelihood of snacking on less nutritious options. Fibre also helps control blood sugar levels and cholesterol and protects against certain types of cancer. It can also play a massive role in how you feel, not just physically but mentally too, as it can impact your digestion, energy levels and productivity.

Where do you find fibre? Many whole grains, fruits, vegetables, and legumes are packed with it. Examples are cauliflower, raspberries, apples, avocados, broad beans and collard greens. So, these are easy additions regardless of most dietary requirements.

Now, if you're wondering how many servings of fruit and vegetables you should aim for daily and you're finding the current suggestion of 5 a day to be a little overwhelming—then aiming for 3 a day could be a great option and starting point.

So, next time you're at the grocery store, consider adding some fibre sources to your list of purchases.

The Importance of Hydration: Not Just About Quenching Thirst

Consider this: humans can survive far longer without food than without water. That's because water is fundamental to all life. So, after proteins and fibre, let's not forget hydration—because the importance of water goes far beyond just "feeling thirsty".

Without it, or with minimal, you'll have trouble strength training, hiking, focusing, or even having good-quality skin.

Reflecting on my exchange year in the U.S. state of Vermont brings this into focus.

Amidst the excitement of leaving my European bubble for the first time, new friends, a strong interest towards my English accent, and many stereotypical American college parties, my usual health habits began to slip in several ways. One was that I often found myself dehydrated, not just from the repetitive less-than-ideal food choices on campus but also from the frequent alcohol and weed use. My gym visits were consistent, but without a clear plan, I was going through the motions rather than progressing.

After several months of this, I noticed a significant weight drop. Stepping on the scale, I saw I was the lightest I'd been in my adult life at 68.5kg. I know this is a chat about fat loss, but it's also about health, and it got to the point in Vermont where I could feel the lack of energy and strength from being at such a relatively light body weight.

That scale weight low was a wake-up call.

Despite enjoying the thrills of student life in the USA, that moment got my butt into gear. I started to re-prioritise my health by making simple but effective choices, such as increasing my water intake. It's a small daily action that significantly impacts overall well-being—even today.

Once I started paying attention to this, I encountered a noticeable trend— many people live in a state of chronic dehydration without even realising it. This chronic dehydration might happen for so long that it subtly establishes itself as your 'new normal,' where the tell-tale signs of thirst become something you're used to. As a result, you might be drinking far less water than you think.

But here's the good news: increasing your water intake is one of the easiest yet most impactful changes you can make for your well-being. Yet, it's frequently overlooked because it lacks the sexiness or marketing buzz of other health trends. So, I have a simple yet essential request: as we finish this chat on hydration, take a moment to pour yourself a glass of water and drink it. It's a small action, but it'll move you one step forward on your health journey.

A general guideline is to aim for at least 8 glasses of water daily, but remember, your personal needs may vary, especially if you're physically active, sweat a lot or live in a warmer climate. Staying hydrated is also about listening to your body and adjusting your water intake to match your lifestyle and physical demands.

On that note, let's discuss the importance of low-calorie-density foods, which, along with drinking more water, should be your focus regarding weight management.

The Importance of Low-Calorie Density Foods

When you're on a journey to lose weight, one of the biggest challenges can be managing hunger while remaining within a calorie deficit. The secret? It's about choosing foods that keep you full and satisfied without going overboard with calories.

Meaning let's talk about low-calorie density foods.

What are these, you ask? They're foods that let you enjoy larger portions but with fewer calories. I'm talking various fruits, veggies, whole grains, and lean proteins. These foods are nutritious, satisfying and low in calorie density.

Take watermelon, for example. You can eat up to 670 grams for just about 200 calories. *That's a massive bowl without the calorie burden.* Then there's tuna, an incredible source of lean protein that can be prepared in many delicious ways. It boosts your protein intake without piling on the calories. Other suggestions are Greek yoghurt, strawberries, oats, spinach, raspberries, blueberries, chicken breast, peppers, and blackberries.

For example, a plate filled with vegetables, a serving of basmati rice, and delicious grilled seasoned chicken or tofu will keep you full and happy while keeping you on track with your health goals. Unlike the bodybuilding stereotype of living on plain chicken and broccoli, eating smart means enjoying decent portions without compromising taste or nutrition.

This talk on low-calorie-dense foods nicely brings up the next section, potential food swaps you can consider on a fat loss journey.

Sensible Food Swaps

In the previous section, we discussed opting for foods with lower calorie density as part of a smart strategy for fat loss. However, it's one thing to suggest these foods, but it's much more helpful to show you exactly how to put them into practice.

Reflecting on my own experience of losing about 20 kg of body fat while living in South London was pivotal in creating this list. It marked the first time I actively learned to maintain a calorie deficit, a previously foreign concept. The food swaps I discovered during that period have become a lasting part of my "calorie deficit dietary habits", and I'll reintroduce a few if I ever feel the need.

So, here's a list of practical food swaps and dining tips that have helped me and many of my 1-2-1 online fitness members. These suggestions could help nudge you towards achieving a calorie deficit:

- Opt for leaner protein sources, such as minced beef with 5% fat instead of 20%.
- Use a one-calorie oil spray instead of traditional cooking oils or butter.
- Opt for low-sugar ketchup rather than the regular kind.
- Select light mayo instead of the full-fat version.
- Pour semi-skimmed or 0% fat milk rather than whole milk.
- Sip on diet soft drinks as opposed to sugary ones. As far as current knowledge, artificial sweeteners are fine in moderation. Enjoying a can of zero-calorie diet soda instead of its sugary counterpart makes much more sense from a fat loss perspective.
- Enjoy low-fat cheese over the full-fat counterpart.
- Scoop up some 0% fat Greek yoghurt instead of the standard option.
- Replace a regular bagel with a bagel thin.
- Boil or air fry foods as a low-calorie alternative to frying in oil or butter.
- Drink your coffee black or with low-fat milk.
- Cut down to 0 or 1 teaspoon of sugar in your coffee, instead of 2 to 4.
- Favour lean meats like turkey and chicken over higher-fat meats.
- If ordering takeout, go for smaller portions.
- Consider miso soup as a low-calorie snack or starter.
- When choosing drinks, consider sticking to water. Cold sparkling water with a wedge of lemon is my preferred option when eating out.

- Aim for about 30 grams of protein in every meal or one portion the size of your palm.
- Make sure to get at least 3 portions of fruits and vegetables daily.
- If you usually have 2 servings of something, try just one.
- Choose air-popped popcorn over chips or buttered popcorn.
- Select thinner crusts or whole wheat crusts for pizza.

Remember, this isn't a be-all and end-all list, nor a strict set of rules you must follow—because attempting to follow all of these could be overwhelming. And yes, losing weight without making all these changes is possible.

However, adopting even a few of these suggestions could significantly help your fat loss efforts. While they seem minor individually, if you do a bunch together, these swaps can make being in a calorie deficit much more manageable.

With a better understanding of potential food swaps and low-calorie density foods, let's discuss supplements—a subject I was unsure about including.

Supplements

Given the ever-growing popularity of supplements, fuelled by advancements in science and savvy marketing, it's worth briefly discussing this topic. Here's a straightforward breakdown of my perspective of things at the time of having this chat:

Gym supplements that are worth it:

- **Protein powders:** Particularly whey protein if you can stomach it, offering high-quality protein for convenience if necessary.

- **Creatine monohydrate:** Extensively researched, it offers various benefits without downsides.
- **Caffeine:** Pre-workouts are overrated, in my opinion. I prefer having a good cup of coffee to help fuel my morning or midday sessions.

Gym supplements that may be worth it:

- **Omega 3:** While some debate its effectiveness, the potential benefits can outweigh the cost, especially when compared to something people won't think twice about paying for—like a round of cocktails.
- **Multivitamins:** Similar to Omega 3s, they can provide a safety net for your nutritional intake.
- **Vitamin D:** This is handy in regions with limited sunlight, like the north of England, or scorching climates discouraging outdoor activities, such as the Alentejo region in Portugal during the summer. In this region, I experienced an astonishing 45 degrees Celsius, which resulted in me barely leaving the comfort of my room.

Gym supplements that you don't need to worry about:

- Everything else I haven't mentioned, and yes, that includes BCAA supplements.

This discussion about everything nutrition-related sets us up nicely for nutrition strategies you can consider following. So, let's get stuck in.

Chapter 3:
Nutrition Strategies

While we continue our conversation about nutrition, I'd like to share a few nutritional approaches you can pick from. I've gathered these strategies over my years of coaching, tailored to fit different readiness levels and lifestyles. Here they are:

Calorie Tracking

Is tracking your calories worth the hassle in the long run? If it's your first time tracking, it's absolutely worth it. It's one of the most accurate ways to understand and manage your nutrition.

I remember being 17 years old and shocked to learn the calorie content of foods like coconut oil, peanut butter, and granola—foods that had been recommended for fat loss. This eye-opener made me realise just how important awareness is when it comes to nutrition, and calorie tracking is the tool that provides this awareness.

Now, I know what you're thinking: "But tracking calories is such a chore, Leo!" Trust me, it might feel tedious at first, but like any new habit, it gets easier with practice. Stick with it, and soon it'll become second nature. Just a few minutes a day is a small price to pay for significant progress toward your fat loss goals.

If you're new to calorie tracking, I recommend committing to it for 30 days—really commit, not just on the days it suits you. This month-long experiment will likely bring some surprising insights about your habits. Start by focusing on tracking calories and protein, as these are the most important for fat loss. Tracking carbohydrates and fats isn't necessary, but if you want to do those and eventually find tracking effortless, go for it.

A common counter-argument I often hear is that tracking can feel obsessive, but I see it differently.

Think of calorie tracking like budgeting for your finances. If you want to improve your financial health, you'd track income and expenses. It's not obsessive; *it's smart*. Similarly, tracking your calories helps you make informed decisions and bring awareness. You'll start asking yourself, "Is this food worth the calorie cost?" or "How does the protein content compare to the calories?"

Tracking teaches you about your habits, while aiming for specific daily targets helps modify those habits to achieve a goal. Many people skip the learning phase and jump straight into rigid targets, which can sometimes lead to frustration. Tracking is a skill. You'll make mistakes, learn about foods, understand your habits, and gradually improve.

Once you're ready to set daily targets, here's what you need to know:

Your calorie deficit goal is key to fat loss, a simple formula to figure this out is to multiply your goal body weight (in pounds) by 11 if you get under 10,000 steps a day, or by 12 if you get over. For instance, if your goal weight is 160lbs and you get over 10,000 steps daily, your calorie goal would be roughly 1,920.

Once you've done the maths, you may think your starting calorie goal is too high, but I can confirm that it is not. The reason you might believe it's too high is that you've historically eaten way too little when trying to lose weight—which is often why you end up overeating and eventually regaining the weight.

Remember, this formula isn't perfect either. Calorie formulas never are—think of them as rough estimates, as the human body is complex. The important thing is that you at least give it a go and be consistent with it for 3 weeks, and then potentially adjust it from there if necessary. Also, don't overthink your goal body weight. It's simply a figure needed for the equation, nothing more—don't get attached to it.

Alternatively, you can check out my free calorie calculator at kairos. online/calorie-calculator to determine your calorie deficit goal.

Whatever your calorie goal, it's helpful to establish a range. Instead of aiming for exactly 1,920 calories, aim for a range of 1,820 to 2,020 to accommodate natural appetite fluctuations. This makes staying consistent easier and helps reduce the pressure of exact numbers.

To make tracking as effective as possible, it's essential to use the right tools:

- **Digital App**: Use a reliable app to accurately track your intake. This will be far more effective and less stressful than keeping a mental tally.
- **Measuring Tools**: Precision is crucial in the beginning, so use a jug and scales to measure food accurately. Weigh your food raw, as cooking changes its weight, making it difficult to be precise.

Initially approaching your calorie intake without accurately tracking, and solely guesstimating, is like playing chess without understanding each piece's strengths and weaknesses. You might make a good move here and there, but without strategic insight, it's all guesswork. Consistent and accurate calorie tracking is like learning the ins and outs of chess strategy—it gives you a deeper understanding of each decision's impact.

It's also crucial to consistently track your food and drink intake every day, not just when it feels convenient. Some people say they don't see progress with food tracking, but often it turns out they skip weekends, forget to log alcohol, overlook cooking oils or butter, miss meals eaten out, or they track sporadically—diligent for a week, then slack on it for the next two. Consider this: calorie tracking feels most tedious when you're about to do something that makes accomplishing your fat loss goals more challenging.

So, if you're ready to gain control over your diet, consider calorie tracking. It might just be the tool you need for a more effective and informed approach to fat loss. However, if you have a history of disordered eating, then I'd be cautious about calorie tracking.

With calorie tracking covered, let's move on to calorie cycling.

Calorie Cycling

So, what is calorie cycling? Instead of following the same daily calorie deficit goal, calorie cycling involves intentionally having higher and lower calorie days throughout the week. Calorie cycling is an adaptable strategy for calorie tracking—it's not a standalone nutrition approach.

One of the best examples illustrating how effective calorie cycling can be is my 1-2-1 online fitness member, good friend, and big Benfica fan, Alex.

When we started working together, Alex had no trouble hitting his nutrition goals during the week but found it challenging to maintain his calorie goals during weekends, when he liked to party and enjoy beer and food with friends. So, we used calorie cycling to accommodate his lifestyle while aiming for fat loss.

To illustrate further, let's revisit the daily goal of 1,920 calories. This amounts to 13,440 calories over a week.

In this situation, Alex and I allocated 2,400 calories for his Saturday and Sunday, then reduced his weekday intake to 1,730, *leaving him consistent with the same 13,440-calorie target.*

With the assistance of calorie cycling, Alex lost 8kg of body fat, got stronger than ever, and made tremendous progress overall—opting to stick with calorie cycling for well over 2 years of working together.

Alternatively, you could try other approaches, too. For example, if you find you're hungrier on workout days and exercise 4 times a week, let's say Monday, Tuesday, Thursday, and Friday, rather than having your higher-calorie days solely on weekends, you could adjust your intake to 2,100 calories on the days you train and 1,680 on rest days. This flexibility makes calorie cycling appealing for managing different daily needs, whether due to work dinners, family gatherings, or a fluctuating appetite.

Of course, you don't have to implement calorie cycling, as you might find it easier to have the same daily goal—which works great for some people, especially those with a more consistent schedule and appetite. However, many other people also find calorie cycling effective and have had great success, including some of my 1-2-1 online fitness members.

Consider giving it a try and see if it suits you.

That said, there's another potential approach you could consider while tracking your calories—the jab deficit.

The Jab Deficit

Going into your calorie deficit and feeling like you'll have to be in it indefinitely can be daunting, giving you the impression that there's no end in sight. This is where the "Jab Deficit" strategy becomes beneficial. It's designed for losing body fat without the intimidating prospect of what feels like a never-ending calorie deficit. The approach involves alternating between a calorie deficit for a set period, such as 2 or 3 weeks, followed by an equal time in maintenance mode, and then cycling between the 2.

This cycling approach makes the process feel more sustainable and can boost your workout sessions, which can sometimes feel more gruelling during prolonged calorie deficits. While the pace of fat loss with a jab deficit is slower than a more consistent calorie deficit, it offers an alternative, especially if you're not under pressure to lose weight quickly for health reasons. However, be prepared for your scale weight to temporarily spike during maintenance phases and know that this is a normal part of the process, not a setback—because there'll still be a downward trend in the long-term.

The jab deficit approach isn't about taking one step back for every two steps forward; instead, it's about taking two steps forward, pausing to stabilise, and then taking two steps forward again.

If you're not interested in calorie tracking, other methods might suit your needs, like the three-plate and two-snack approach we're about to cover.

Three Plates and Two Snacks Approach

The 'Three Plates and Two Snacks' approach is straightforward for structuring meals. It's perfect if you're going through a phase of your life in which calorie counting isn't possible, you're not ready for it yet, or you're just looking for an easy-to-follow eating routine.

The Concept: You'll have three main meals and two snacks daily.

Your Plates: Each of your 3 meals should be the following:

- **Half of Your Plate—Vegetables or Salad:** Fill this part with colourful, fibre-rich veggies. Think sauteed red cabbage, steamed broccoli, or a fresh salad.
- **One Quarter—Protein:** This is your fullness and recovery booster. Choose from meats, fish, eggs, or plant-based options like lentils or tofu.
- **Last Quarter—Carbohydrates or Fats:** You could choose carbohydrates such as potatoes and rice or healthy fats like avocado slices.

Snacking: Your 2 snacks are opportunities for nutritional boosts. You could pick from a piece of fruit, a vegetable or a protein source that fits into the palm of your hand. This will further help with convenience and reduce hunger throughout the day.

Why It's a Winning Strategy: This approach isn't just about what you eat; it's about developing a sustainable habit. It's structured enough to guide you but flexible enough to fit into any lifestyle. Whether you're a busy professional, a student, or someone juggling multiple roles, this method adapts to your life. So, by following the 'Three Plates and 2 Snacks' approach, you're taking a big step towards balanced eating.

However, if you feel this approach isn't right for you either, let's discuss the hand-size portion guide.

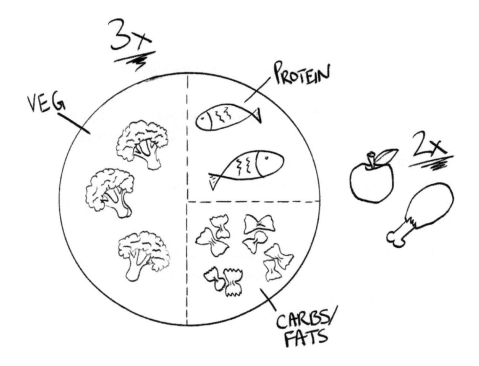

The Hand-Size Portion Guide

The hand-size portion guide is a handy way to determine how much you should eat. It is tailored just for you because it uses your hands to measure food.

Here's how to use it:

- For protein, like chicken or fish, use the palm of your hand. The size and thickness of your palm give you a good idea of the right amount, usually between 85-150g.
- Use a cupped hand to get the right portion of carbs like rice, pasta, or potatoes.
- For fats like nuts or cheese, your thumb is your guide. It represents about a tablespoon.

- For oils and butter, the tip of your thumb is just right for a teaspoon.
- The amount for veggies, like carrots or salad, is a fist-size.

Remember, like any other method, this method isn't perfect, and you might need to tweak it. If you're feeling too full or not losing weight after 3 weeks, you might need to cut back a bit. On the flip side, adding a little more to your plate is okay if you're always hungry and losing weight too fast.

With that covered, let's move on to what's personally a less favoured but too popular approach to ignore—meal plans.

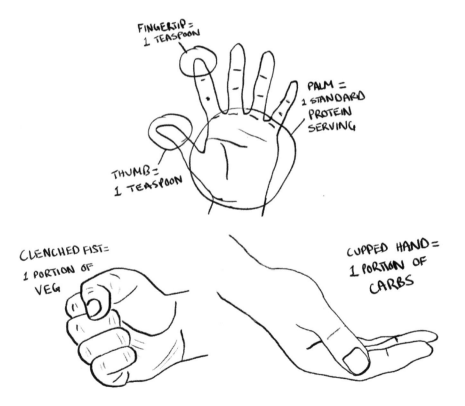

Meal Planning

Let me take you back to my days as a personal trainer on the gym floor. I was chatting with one of my new clients, Aisling, a busy professional from Ireland. After a few weeks together, she pulled out a meal plan she'd once paid dearly for, full of very specific foods, precise serving sizes, and timings for each meal and snack.

But here's where it got tricky: as a mother of two and a professional with demanding hours, Aisling found it virtually impossible to stick to this rigid schedule. It wasn't about "a lack of willpower." The reality was that a meal plan that dictated what to eat, when, and how much to eat just wasn't feasible for someone with her lifestyle. Ironically, she didn't even like some of the foods listed.

This experience highlighted a critical flaw in such meal plans—they often seem more designed to make quick money for the providers than to offer real, sustainable help to their users. While a prescribed meal plan might seem initially appealing, I've come to see rigid meal plans that leave no room for personal preference or life's unpredictable moments as unhelpful and setting people up for failure.

Consider the nature of life—unexpected birthday parties, spontaneous barbecues with friends, and co-workers' weddings. What do you do when these events arise? You might be at a loss if you always follow a strict meal plan. The dependency of always having a meal plan telling you exactly what to do is precisely where meal plans fall short.

They don't empower you with the knowledge of 'how' and 'why'—the essential tools for making informed decisions or the ins and outs of achieving your goals.

It's like the old saying: Give a man a fish, and you feed him for a day—that's a meal plan. Teach a man to fish, and you feed him for a lifetime. That's understanding the principles of energy balance and food quality—which I did with Aisling.

This understanding equips you for lifelong success, allowing you to navigate everyday life's unpredictability.

With my beliefs on meal planning now shared, let's move on to a nutritional approach that must be discussed within this chapter—intuitive eating.

Intuitive Eating

Intuitive eating is sometimes mistaken for a fat loss diet, but it is not. Its philosophy promotes a healthy attitude toward food and body image. It focuses on eating in response to your body's hunger cues and stopping when full. This approach emphasises listening to and trusting your body's signals rather than following external dietary rules or restrictions.

From my perspective, the ideal place to be, nutrition-wise, is one where we, including you and me, are in tune with our body's hunger and fullness cues. However, achieving this state might be challenging if you've historically struggled with nutrition.

This is because intuitive eating, like any skill, requires a certain level of proficiency and experience that must be developed over time. It's unlikely someone can overcome years of nutritional challenges, societal pressures, and a skewed relationship with food and suddenly wake up able to intuitively understand their body's needs.

If you find intuitive eating difficult after a history of dieting struggles, consider this: you might need a "preparatory phase." This could involve a period of consistently tracking your food intake or following other structured guidelines, such as the ones mentioned earlier. These strategies can serve as stepping stones toward intuitive eating. By applying these methods consistently, you gradually build experience and knowledge about your daily food choices, making the transition to a more intuitive approach much smoother.

I want to clarify that I am not against intuitive eating; it should be the ultimate goal for everyone's eating habits. However, my words were more of a warning against viewing it as a straightforward solution if you've been caught in a cycle of dieting struggles for years or even decades. Although long-term, with patience and practice, you can successfully adopt intuitive eating.

Overall, by being consistent with nutrition approaches such as calorie tracking, 3 plates 2 snacks, or the hand-sized portion guide, and then sticking to it with about 85-95% consistency and being mindful of the guidelines and suggestions from the meal planning and intuitive eating parts, you're really setting yourself up for your success.

Now, you might wonder, why not aim for 100%? Here's the thing: striving for absolute perfection in your fitness and diet regimen isn't just unrealistic; it's unnecessary. It's essential to make these approaches work for you, fitting seamlessly into your life rather than becoming a massive source of stress or taking over entirely. Fitness should improve your life and make it more enjoyable, not take away from it.

With sustainability and consistency in mind, let's touch on the polar opposite—aggressive fat loss approaches.

Aggressive Fat Loss Approaches

Does this scenario ring a bell? You've spent the past few months or years enjoying life to the fullest, indulging more and exercising less. Initially, you're not bothered by it, mainly because you're having fun. But then, the moment of truth arrives when your favourite t-shirt feels uncomfortably tight, reinforcing the fact that your lifestyle choices are starting to catch up to you.

In a rush to shed the extra weight, you opt for the quickest, most aggressive fat loss strategies. After all, who has time to waste? Plus, you're eager to see immediate results.

I get where you're coming from with this approach. However, typical aggressive methods often lead to frustration and a pattern of yo-yo dieting. Initially, you might see dramatic weight loss, which fuels your motivation to keep going. But soon, the intensity of your weight loss plan catches up with you. Energy levels plummet, workouts become a chore, and overwhelming hunger pangs lead to binge eating, erasing all your progress and leaving you back at square one.

My stance with aggressive fat loss phases has evolved over my coaching career. While I used to oppose them, I now see their potential benefit in specific scenarios, particularly at the start of a fat loss journey when motivation is typically at its highest and there's a lot of body fat to lose for health reasons. Aggressive dieting might also be a good option if you feel you need to see rapid results to want to keep going. Still, it's not suitable for everyone—I'd only recommend aggressive fat loss approaches if you have at least 15kg or 33lbs to lose.

If you're considering this route to address health concerns and need to lose significant weight quickly, an aggressive approach could potentially be a brief solution. *However, this requires near-perfect adherence for about a month.* Remember, this phase will be challenging; it's meant to be intense and is not a long-term solution. Commit to this approach only if you're prepared for the rigour and are ready to switch to a more sustainable plan at the end of week 4.

Limiting this phase to no more than a month is crucial to avoid burnout and continue long-term progress.

A potential calorie deficit formula for your brief, aggressive approach consists of using your goal body weight as part of the equation. Start by multiplying your goal body weight from anywhere between 6 to 12, then add one each week. However, I would not recommend multiplying it by 6 as that is extremely aggressive. The more body fat you have to lose, the lower you could potentially go with your deficit. I feel most comfortable starting at 7 or 8 for aggressive phases—depending on the starting point and the goal body weight.

I'll provide an example below, using a random goal bodyweight of 180lbs to determine what someone might aim for within their first few weeks:

- Week 1: 180lbs times by 7 = 1,260 calories daily
- Week 2: 180lbs times by 8 = 1,440 calories daily
- Week 3: 180lbs times by 9 = 1,620 calories daily
- Week 4: 180lbs times by 10 = 1,800 calories daily
- Week 5: Return to a slight calorie deficit which you can determine via my calorie calculator kairos.online/calorie-calculator

Throughout the first 4 weeks, you'll also do your best to hit your daily protein goal while ensuring that healthy fats make up about 25% of your daily caloric intake—because fats are crucial for health.

The mistake many people make, potentially you included, is continuing with the aggressive calorie deficit beyond the first 4 weeks due to the excitement with the rapid drops in weight. Do not do this. You are not an exception, no matter how much of a special fairy you think you are. You'll still lose weight while being in a sustainable calorie deficit—after all, it's a deficit. However, it'll be at a pace that'll allow you to keep going and not continue to take over every waking moment of your life.

It's also vital that you do not go lower than 50% of your maintenance calories at any point. So, if any of the above equations are to give you a calorie deficit goal lower than 50% of your maintenance calories, you would stick with the 50% goal instead, slowly increasing it from there following the above formula. This will help prevent the pitfalls of being overly aggressive to the point it'll do more harm. You could also use my free calorie calculator to help you figure out your maintenance calories.

Remember, aggressiveness only works short-term, and many people fall short because they try to stick with it for too long, which causes them to continuously go around in circles. Understand that in the long-term, there's no fast or slow way to lose weight; there's only a right and wrong way. This fitness thing is a lifelong journey—and eventually, you'll be forced to treat it like one for results that stick.

Now, let's focus on another crucial aspect regarding food exclusions. This involves understanding the result of completely cutting out certain foods from your diet. It's an important topic, as it happens often, and making these overly restrictive choices can usually lead to challenges down the line.

The Myth of Exclusion

Before starting her fitness journey with me as a 1-2-1 online fitness member, Sewa, a part-time university student practising medicine, from South London, believed she needed to cut out various foods entirely and follow strict meal instructions on what to eat, when, and how.

Imagine her surprise when I told her the opposite: 'Nothing is off-limits.'

'Nothing? Are you sure?' she asked, bewildered.

Now, saying 'nothing is off-limits' doesn't mean there are no limits—there's a difference.

But consider this: If I say, 'Don't think of a pink elephant,' what pops into your mind? I'd go all-in on a poker game that it's a pink elephant.

This paradox explains why strict dietary restrictions often fail. It's the same way that telling yourself that you can't have sugar, carbs, processed foods, bread, fried foods, white rice, and so on might work in the short-term, but over time, you'll likely find this approach more challenging. This restrictive mindset was partly why Sewa had previously found herself going in circles with her fitness goals prior to working with me.

In the weight loss world, there's a persistent myth that the more foods you exclude from your diet, the better your health and fat loss results will be. This belief is behind the popularity of dietary approaches like paleo, keto, and carnivore diets. But let's set allergies, health conditions, and intolerances aside for a moment—because excluding certain foods for these reasons may make sense for your physical well-being.

Regarding general fat loss, this exclusion mindset might hamper your progress.

Here's a mindset shift, that worked tremendously for Sewa and got her incredible results, that could be a game-changer for you, too: Instead of fixating on what you should eliminate, focus on what you can *add* to your diet. Consider including more water and single-ingredient foods like protein, vegetables, fruits, and fibre. This shift towards inclusion means you naturally start eating more nutritious foods.

Plus, here's the best part: You'll likely feel too satisfied to overeat the less nutritious options you'd typically cut out—not because you're forcing exclusion, but because your body feels more satisfied with everything you should focus on anyway.

Embracing an inclusion mindset, where you focus on adding beneficial foods rather than strictly cutting everything you perceive to be "bad" out, tends to be more sustainable and easier to maintain. This approach is healthier for your body and mind and more realistic for your lifestyle, making it more likely for you to stay consistent and see real, lasting results.

Now that we've discussed food exclusions and inclusions, let's touch on the final 2 nutrition-related topics—cravings and alcohol. Starting with cravings.

Dealing with Cravings

Before diving into cravings, you must understand that cravings are entirely normal. You're not unusual, different or strange for having them—it's a part of being human.

Now, aside from being human, which other potential reasons cause cravings? One significant reason is the involvement of large food corporations. They invest millions into food engineering, using top scientists and experts to enhance foods' taste, aroma, and texture. These adjustments are designed to make it harder for you to stop eating, ultimately boosting their profits.

This isn't to alarm you but to raise awareness.

Now, let's explore effective strategies to manage cravings.

First and foremost, no food should be entirely off-limits, echoing what we discussed in "The Myth of Exclusion" section. Restricting yourself too much often increases cravings in the long-term. However, this doesn't mean there shouldn't be boundaries, as moderation is key.

A good suggestion could be the '20-minute rule.' When a craving hits, allow yourself to have the desired food, but wait for 20 minutes first. You'll often find that the craving passes after 20 minutes, indicating that it may have been a momentary urge rather than genuine hunger.

Then there's 'The Apple Test.' Ask yourself if you're hungry enough to eat an apple. If not, your craving might stem from boredom rather than hunger. If yes, eat an apple first, which might curb your initial craving.

Another helpful concept is setting 'Bright Lines,' which are personal rules you commit to following. For instance, my bright line is that if I want dessert after a meal, I must first eat a piece of fruit. No fruit, no dessert. This is a personal rule I've followed for years. Establishing a clearly laid out bright line can help with your eating habits. I'll touch more on bright lines later.

If you find you're often "giving in to cravings," I'd suggest not skipping meals. Skipping meals might escalate hunger to a point where it becomes difficult to control, leading to overindulgence in cravings. This can result in a cycle of meal skipping and binge eating, which is counterproductive to managing cravings and making fat loss progress.

Lastly, and perhaps most importantly, overcoming your craving might be as simple as enjoying some of what you've been craving. So, perhaps have some chocolate and move on with your life.

With these strategies and thought processes, you can navigate your cravings more effectively.

Now, let's turn our attention to the final crucial topic in this part of our chat: alcohol and its impact on fat loss.

Alcohol and Fat Loss

Right from the start, I promised to keep things 100% real with you. So, let's address one of the most socially acceptable yet potentially detrimental habits when it comes to fitness and fat loss: alcohol consumption.

It's somewhat ironic—many are quick to criticise foods like bread, white rice, or artificial sweeteners, yet often overlook the impacts of alcohol. I'm no stranger to it either; my late teens into my early twenties were marked by memorable parties involving plenty of alcohol in South London, Burlington, and Ottawa.

This isn't about dictating your choices—I'm not here to do that. There's no denying that alcohol can be a great social lubricant. Plus, you're an adult, and you can make your own decisions. My goal is to provide you with honest thoughts so you can make informed choices about alcohol, especially if you're trying to lose fat.

If you rarely or never drink, this alcohol chat might not be relevant. But if you enjoy the occasional drink, let's expand on how alcohol can affect your fat loss efforts.

Here are a few commonly asked questions:

- Can you enjoy a drink and stay on track with your fat loss goals?
- How does alcohol fit into a healthy lifestyle?
- Do I have to ban it completely?

First, it's helpful to understand that alcohol has calories—7 calories per gram, to be precise. Whether a pint of beer, a glass of wine, or a cocktail, each drink contributes to your daily calorie intake. But here's the important part: the impact of alcohol isn't just about the calories in your glass. It's also about how it influences your food choices and appetite.

For example, have you ever noticed how a fun night out can transform into a spontaneous feast, be it takeaway or late-night snacks? Alcohol has a way of boosting what I like to informally call the 'fuck it factor', where suddenly, the greasy takeaway pizza and the oil-drenched fried chicken seem irresistible—and because your decision-making is a bit more relaxed, overeating becomes too easy.

It's common for a night of drinking to send your daily calories soaring, especially when you factor in the rounds of drinks followed by the unplanned fast-food run.

But here's the good news: enjoying alcohol doesn't have to be a no-go. It's about finding a happy medium, a way to enjoy your drink without throwing your fat loss goals off track. For example, consider preparing in advance the next time you plan to enjoy a drink or 2. If you know you'll be out for the night, consider adjusting your calories earlier in the day to accommodate the extra intake. Or, if you're following the 3 plates, 2 snacks approach, as previously mentioned, you could balance your day by swapping a snack for a drink or both snacks for 2 drinks.

It's about making room for enjoyment without overdoing it because planning is vital.

Enjoying a drink now and then is part of life for many people. With some planning, it doesn't have to derail your health and fitness journey. However, if drinking is a daily or near-daily habit, it could be worth recognising that it might be a major factor holding you back from progress. In that case, it's worth considering whether it's time to step back.

Overall, before moving on to the next section of "Everyday Movement," I want to highlight one last thing—whichever nutrition approach you pick from the above options, ensure that you at least give it a fair shot. Trying it for 1 or 2 days and then stopping is not giving yourself a chance.

An example is when I began Brazilian Jiu-Jitsu, I paid for a three-month membership upfront. This commitment ensured that I gave myself ample time to immerse myself in the sport, understand its nuances a little better, and truly assess my enjoyment.

You don't need to stick at it for 3 months. It could be just a couple of weeks. But often, our initial discomfort or struggle gives way to growth and enjoyment, but only if we give ourselves the time to experience and overcome these early challenges. If you don't like it after giving it a fair shot, find an alternative. But it's about giving the new endeavour a fair chance to become a meaningful part of your life before making a definitive judgement.

Chapter 4:
Everyday Movement

Sipping on our hot cups, let's explore the everyday movements that significantly contribute to fat loss. Strength training is essential, and we'll discuss that in more depth later. But for now, we'll talk about Non-Exercise Activity Thermogenesis (NEAT), walking, hobbies, and a sprinkle of Norwegian wisdom.

NEAT: A Cornerstone of Fat Loss

First, your NEAT is your everyday movement outside of conscious exercise. NEAT consists of all those small activities you might not think much about: walking up and down stairs, gardening, carrying shopping bags, pacing during phone calls, or house chores. These activities, with a calorie deficit, boost your fat loss progress.

You might be surprised to learn that NEAT plays a pivotal role in sustainable fat loss. But think about it like this: a week has 168 hours. If you're getting 7 hours of sleep each night, that's 49 hours per week spent asleep. This leaves 119 waking hours. Now, let's be generous and say you exercise more than the average person, and imagine you're doing 4 weekly sessions for an hour and a half each. That's 6 hours dedicated to exercise, leaving 113 hours unaccounted for.

A common misconception about fat loss is overestimating the impact of these 6 hours of exercise while neglecting the other 113 hours. I understand you're busy. However, if, for example, during those 113 hours, you're predominantly sedentary—sitting at a desk, driving, or relaxing on the internet—you're missing out on massive opportunities to boost your fat loss.

While exercise has numerous benefits, it can only do so much for fat loss, especially if most of your time is spent stationary. This is where the importance of NEAT becomes noticeable–what you'll be doing within many of those 113 hours makes the difference.

This discussion of NEAT naturally leads to an often-overlooked yet vital topic: walking. Let's explore how this simple activity can significantly improve your fat loss journey.

The Power of Walking

In my early teens, specifically during 'Activities Week' at Dunraven Secondary School in South London, I was assigned to a group focused on walking through the English countryside on foot. This was given to me because I missed the sign-up deadline for Activities Week, meaning I missed out on the more popular physical activities that teenagers in London would generally be more interested in, such as football, basketball or martial arts.

The switch to long daily walks in the countryside was unlike my usual routine, typically consisting of playing video games, texting, or hanging out with friends around South London.

Initially, the prospect of spending days walking seemed dull, especially compared to my mates who were playing football. However, this led to an unexpected revelation. The countryside walks opened up a new world of physical activity and mental stimulation I hadn't known before. My daily step count at least tripled, and without even focusing on dieting or fat loss, I noticed a significant positive change in my physical health and mental well-being, which was only helped by the social connections formed with others on the walks. That's when a young Leo forever learned about the power of walking.

Two weeks later, I also noticed a significant drop in the scale for the first time in a long time.

Realise that walking is an incredibly straightforward and effective form of exercise. I know many people who have lost a massive amount of body fat simply because they added more walking to their routine—and that was their only form of exercise. Getting extra steps in is something I'd recommend you do, too, especially if you're averaging less than 5,000 steps daily. Regular walking improves heart health, mood, and even cognitive function. Plus, it's an ideal starting point if you're new to exercise or returning after a break.

To make walking a habit, start with small, achievable goals, like a 15-minute walk during lunch or choosing stairs over elevators. Then, gradually increase your steps until you reach a point you feel you can consistently sustain. For example, whenever I start with a new 1-2-1 online fitness member, I might get them to aim for 2,500 more than their recent average. So, say they'd recently been averaging 5,500 steps before starting with me; their new goal would be 8,000 steps per day. A great way to make your walks more enjoyable is with podcasts (The Leo Alves Podcast, in case you're curious), music, or overdue catch-ups with old friends via a phone call.

That said, walking isn't the only way people move frequently. So, let's explore how other cultures sometimes stay active.

Rediscovering Joy in Movement

Have you heard of the Norwegian concept of "friluftsliv," which means "open-air/outdoor living"? It's about connecting with nature and finding well-being through outdoor activities. While not strictly associated with exercise, it can typically result in outside movement, e.g. hiking, cycling, or even tree climbing.

Then you have "Kenkō Taisō," known as Japanese health exercises. These simple routines, typically stretching and gentle callisthenics, improve overall health. Popular among all ages in Japan, these exercises are often done in groups in parks, promoting physical and social well-being.

I bring these up not to help you on your next pub quiz but because many adults, potentially you included, have entered adulthood with a skewed relationship with movement and exercise. Think back to your school days when exercise was often used as punishment. Whether it was push-ups for the losing team in P.E. or laps around the pitch for misbehaviour, many of us grew up associating exercise with negative experiences. This could explain why, as adults, some of us have a strained relationship with physical activity. It's vital, however, to find a form of movement you enjoy, or hate the least—like the Scandinavians and Japanese. It could be rock climbing, hiking, or martial arts—and aim to make it a regular part of your life.

Time in the Sun

If there's one hugely overlooked factor in life, it's getting outside in the sun more.

Now, I'm aware that everyday movement doesn't necessarily mean spending time in the sun. Nor am I saying that if you feel you have body fat to lose, just sit in the sun, and everything will be sorted. *What I am saying is that it should not be overlooked as an essential part of your lifestyle and overall health.*

Sunlight exposure is essential for Vitamin D, dubbed the "sunshine vitamin." Vitamin D supports bone health, mood regulation, and cardiovascular health. Despite its importance, its deficiency is widespread.

I've noticed significant improvements in my physical and mental well-being in sunnier locations. Whether I was soaking up the sun in Italy or enjoying the brighter days in the Kansai region of Japan, the contrast in how I felt was stark compared to the often gloomy weather in England, one of the significant factors that influenced my decision to move from London.

While I understand that not everyone can easily access sunny weather—like when I briefly visited Reykjavik in November, where daylight was scarce—I suggest seizing the opportunity to be in natural sunlight when possible—even if it's just for 15 minutes a day. If you're in a less sunny location, consider vitamin D supplementation to mimic one of the sun's major benefits.

So, in the nicest way possible—touch grass.

As we transition from discussing everyday movement, cultural wisdom, and sunlight to exploring the role of strength training in your fitness journey, remember that sometimes, the simplest activities can lead to the most significant changes in your health and well-being.

Chapter 5:
The Power of Strength Training

As a teenager, I went for my first gym workout at a place tucked away in Mitcham, South London, with my best mate from school, who was equally as naive about fitness. We went through a chest session inspired by our youthful ignorance and YouTube fitness influencers.

Despite how poor that session might have been (we were clueless), I slowly realised the advantages of strength training over time. Far from making you "overly bulky," inflexible, or prone to injury, the many benefits might surprise you.

So, let's take a deep breath, inhale, and dive into how helpful it can be.

Strength training is magical for your body—increasing muscle mass, bone density, strength, power, and endurance. It doesn't stop there—it also improves motor control (including balance), mobility, and flexibility. Beyond the physical, your resting metabolic rate gets a boost, contributing to a more efficient metabolism.

The perks extend into your cells with autophagy—the body's way of cleaning out damaged cells to regenerate newer, healthier ones. Expect better sleep, heightened self-esteem, and a surge in confidence.

To put it bluntly, it increases your sex appeal, too.

But the good news doesn't end with what strength training adds to your life—it's also about what it takes away. It can help reduce fat, physical fatigue, and risks of insulin resistance and hypertension. It tackles joint pain, sexual dysfunction, and the declines in cognitive health that can come with age. Moreover, it can be helpful against anxiety and depression.

And now, exhale.

This isn't to say that you must look and train like a bodybuilder—unless that's your goal. Nor is it to say that you "must" strength train on a fat loss journey either—because you don't. However, this is all highlighted to help you recognise that a well-rounded strength training routine can be a game-changer for anyone, even if done 2 to 3 times a week and progressively overloaded over time (more on progressive overload later).

Strength training is not just beneficial; it's life-saving, especially when you consider that one of the most common causes of mortality among elderly folks is from falls. To quote Jonathan Goodman, *"My dad has exercised every week since I was young. At 78, he plays with my kids on the floor while many of his friends need assistance. Fitness doesn't seem like it matters until one day, it becomes obvious."*

The likely difference between his dad and his dad's mates? Continued, active use of the body.

If starting a strength training regimen feels daunting, don't worry. The following chat will provide you with practical advice to help kickstart your journey. Believe it or not, it could be the most impactful decision you make for your health.

Strength Training vs. Cardio

Now, you might wonder why our conversation, focused primarily on fat loss, discusses the benefits of strength training rather than cardio, such as running on the treadmill or using the cross trainer, the go-to for many on a fat loss journey.

The truth might surprise you: strength training trumps cardio (walking aside) for long-term fat loss that sticks. Not that it necessarily must be one or the other, but in my opinion, cardio comes low on the list of priorities for sustainably shedding fat.

When I mention that strength training is superior to cardio for fat loss, I'm frequently met with the counterargument: "But cardio burns more calories! How can strength training be better?"

It's a common thought that a cardio session's immediate calorie-burning effect makes it superior. Still, this view doesn't account for the bigger picture and long-term benefits of strength training.

So, with that said, let's expand on why strength training should be your main go-to:

1. **Metabolic Advantages:** Muscle mass is metabolically active, meaning it burns more calories at rest than fat. I'll discuss this further shortly.
2. **Preserving Muscle:** As you lose weight, you must ensure you're shedding fat, not muscle. Strength training helps maintain and even build muscle tissue, ensuring your fat loss is healthy.
3. **Functional Strength:** Increased strength translates to a more effortless daily life. Whether it's carrying groceries, putting your luggage in the overhead cabin, or keeping up with energetic kids, *a*

stronger you means a more active you—taking it back to our discussion on NEAT and its importance for fat loss.

4. **Transferrable Benefits:** The strength you build in the gym empowers you beyond physical fitness. It boosts your confidence and self-esteem, which can help tremendously on a fat loss journey.

Hearing some of the above points may initially sound odd. However, anyone who has committed some time to strength training will echo these sentiments, backing its fantastic impact.

Now, before expanding on fasted cardio and LISS, let me clarify 2 points:

Firstly, strength training should be pursued with the goal of becoming stronger and achieving performance milestones—like nailing that first chin-up or deadlifting your bodyweight—not done for the specific intent of fat loss. You'll then discover fat loss can be a byproduct when aiming for these performance targets—with proper nutrition, of course.

Secondly, *I'm not dismissing the value of cardio.* It's important, too, particularly for your heart health—which, after all, is the most important muscle in the body. It's just that when it comes to fat loss *specifically,* cardio's efficacy is often overrated by many people starting—resulting in the common scenario of feeling like they're on a hamster wheel for months and years of going around in circles with their progress—which is why this "strength training vs. cardio" section is included.

Anyway, let's speak a tad more on cardio before we go in on everything strength training.

Fasted Cardio and LISS

When living in South London, I once had a phase where I did cardio in the form of maximal incline walking on the treadmill, first thing in the morning, always with just a banana and some chocolate milk beforehand. However, the critical aspect of fat loss remained my overall calorie intake, not the timing of my cardio.

When it comes to the effectiveness of fasted cardio for fat loss, the timing—whether you do it fasted or not—doesn't matter. It boils down to personal preference and what you can be most consistent with. If you like eating or drinking a little something before cardio, that's fine. If you prefer to do it on an empty stomach, that's okay too. Like I said, the key to fat loss is maintaining a calorie deficit over time, not whether you did or didn't consume anything before your cardio session.

I'll also say that if you are to do cardio, then low-intensity steady-state (LISS) cardio is an excellent choice for many. It's beneficial for heart health and a fantastic way to increase your daily step count, offering a gentler alternative to high-intensity interval training (HIIT), which I believe is generally a poor idea for fat loss, or running, which can sometimes place a lot of stress through the knee joints depending on how much weight you have to lose. Plus, LISS allows for multitasking, making it an addition that's easier to stick with doing. I'll sometimes watch Japanese language learning videos, last night's football highlights or even video call catch-ups with friends.

With your improved understanding of fasted cardio, LISS, and strength training over cardio specifically for fat loss, let's turn your attention to strength training's metabolic advantages. I'll use a straightforward analogy to help explain this.

Muscle Mass and Metabolism

The next time your mate questions why on Earth you're prioritising your strength training for fat loss, here's an analogy you can impress them with: think of your muscles as engines and your body as a car.

Now, imagine 2 cars: one with a small engine and one with a slightly larger engine. A car with a slightly larger engine will burn more fuel even when idle simply because it has the potential to do more work.

In this analogy, doing strength training is like upgrading your car's engine to a slighter larger one. Even when you're not driving (exercising), your larger engine (muscle mass) requires more fuel (calories) to maintain itself.

So, by increasing your muscle mass through strength training, you're effectively turning your body into a slightly more fuel-hungry machine, increasing your resting metabolic rate and burning more calories every day.

This is why strength training can be more effective for fat loss in the long-term than cardio; it's like constantly running a slightly larger engine, even when you're not actively "driving" it during exercise. Meanwhile, only focusing on cardio will forever leave you with a slightly smaller engine, limiting your calorie burn to only when you're on the move and missing out on the continual, passive calorie burn that a bigger engine provides.

This is also why it's crucial to continue lifting weights and emphasising protein as you go through a fat loss journey—you must send a signal to your body that it needs its muscle, which will help you more in the long run.

However, some might argue, "Aren't the metabolic differences from muscle gain minimal, making little difference?" The metabolic impact of increased muscle is indeed modest—but it all helps. Plus, as mentioned earlier, it's *also* about the benefits that spill into other parts of your life. Remember when I said that more muscle means more strength for everyday activities, making them easier—carrying groceries, lifting luggage, or keeping up with energetic children—which all naturally result in higher levels of NEAT?

Now that we've tackled muscle mass and metabolism, we can smoothly transition to the most efficient ways of building these—compound exercises.

Compound Movements

One spring, during a lengthy bus trip from the capital to southern Portugal, I received a notification on my phone about a request for 1-2-1 online fitness coaching. As I opened the application form, I recognised the name—it was Kaffy.

"Hey Leo, I know it's been about three years since we last worked together, but I really enjoyed our first time and would love to team up again."

Kaffy, from South London, who loves travelling all over Europe and her biscuits, had always been a delightful 1-2-1 online fitness member, so I was happy to welcome her back.

Reviewing her inquiry, Kaffy mentioned her goals were to improve her chin-ups and develop stronger and bigger glutes. She also noted that most of her training sessions needed to be early in the morning before work, and therefore, concise sessions to fit her schedule were a must.

The answer to limited training time? Focus on compound movements.

Now, rest assured, it's essential to understand that developing an 'overly big and bulky' physique is not an automatic outcome. Not strength training because you're worried about becoming "overly big and bulky" is like not wanting to cook in case you accidentally become a master chef.

Achieving a specific look involves a certain type of training, a particular nutritional approach, time, consistency, hard work, and, to some extent, genetics. So, unless that's your focus, you won't magically wake up "too big and bulky" one day.

So focusing primarily on compound movements, like I did with Kaffy, is often the best approach. But what exactly are compound exercises? In resistance training, there are 2 main types of exercises:

- **Compound Exercises:** These involve multiple muscle groups working simultaneously. For example, a barbell bent-over row primarily works the back but also stimulates the biceps, abs, and hamstrings. Similarly, a bodyweight dip targets the chest, shoulders, and triceps.
- **Isolation Exercises:** These target a single muscle group. A dumbbell bicep curl, for instance, focuses solely on the biceps, while a dumbbell side raise works the shoulders.

Understanding this difference clarifies why compound exercises are more efficient for muscle building. They provide more 'bang for your buck' by engaging several muscle groups simultaneously. Think of compound exercises almost like a Swiss Army knife: like how this one tool can handle various tasks, compound exercises allow you to work on multiple muscles at once. This isn't to dismiss the value of isolation exercises—they have their place, especially for targeting specific areas or when you're getting more exhausted towards the end of a workout, as they do not require as much energy as compound lifts. However, compound exercises should be your primary focus for overall progress.

Later in our chat, I'll share example workouts incorporating compound exercises tailored for you. But for now, we must discuss a crucial component of successful strength training: ensuring you get up and go to the gym.

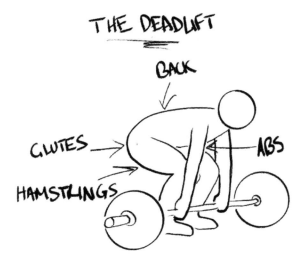

THE DEADLIFT

BACK

GLUTES

ABS

HAMSTRINGS

Tips for Boosting Workout Motivation

Let me share a short story about Igor, a brilliant Brazilian video game developer from South London and one of my 1-2-1 online fitness members. Before we teamed up, Igor struggled with consistency in his workouts, because he'd often stop before gaining any real momentum.

During our initial conversation, Igor asked about ways to boost his workout motivation. I can't recall my exact words as this chat was years ago, but I do remember discussing the fickle nature of motivation itself.

If you've been struggling, it might be because you expect motivation to magically hit you one day.

You might think it works like this:
Motivation → Action → Results → Repeat

In reality, the cycle is often reversed:
Action → Results → Motivation → Repeat

I advised Igor to start by almost 'forcing' himself into action, committing to workouts even when he didn't feel like it. But keep going, and as the results show, it'll fuel your motivation to continue. Remember, consistency breeds results, and results spark motivation. It's a beautiful cycle.

And time proved this right.

After some initial consistency without visible results, Igor texted me one day, ecstatic: 'I can't believe it. I was showering this morning and for the first time ever, I saw my calf muscle!!!!!' Since then, he's made strength training a regular part of his life.

Remember that motivation is a feeling, and feelings come and go. The same way you're not always going to feel happy, sad or angry is the same way you're not always going to feel motivated. However, just because you're not feeling happy, it doesn't mean that you still shouldn't say thank you to the cashier when they scan your groceries, the waiter when he serves your food or that you shouldn't hold the door open for the next person. It's the same way in which just because you don't feel motivated, it doesn't mean you still shouldn't do your workout, go on your walk or eat your vegetables.

You do these things because that's just who you are.

With that deeper understanding in place now, let's walk through some of my favourite tactics to help you stay consistent:

- **Prioritise Your Workouts:** Schedule your workouts before anything else. Treating them as non-negotiable appointments, just like you would for other essential things, lays a foundation for consistency. Waiting until you 'have time' often leads to skipped sessions.

- **Seek Accountability:** Join a community, hire a personal trainer, or find an online coach. The support, teamwork, and guidance remove the guesswork and make your commitment tangible. Plus, you'll have skin in the game when you're paying to have someone in your corner.

- **Change Your Environment:** If gym attendance is sporadic, bring the workouts home. Alternatively, a gym membership could provide a fresh environment to re-spark your routine if home workouts are tedious.

- **Start Small:** Commit to the first 2 exercises on low-motivation days. Often, the hardest part is starting, and if you want to stop after the first 2 exercises, that's fine. However, once you begin, the momentum might carry you through a whole session. It's kinda like when you start reading a book. Once you're a few pages in, you often want to keep going.

- **Embrace it:** There's abundant motivational content out there, but ultimately, action is on you. There comes a time when you need to rise above procrastination and 'do the damn thing'. Your health and journey are your responsibility—no one else's.

Overall, initially getting yourself to show up more will be challenging because you won't feel like it. But if you don't make yourself, no one else will. You're not always motivated to go to work, but you do it because you have to pay your bills. It's your health, journey, and duty. Tough love? Maybe, but it's true.

With workout motivation now covered, let's move on to the last 2 parts of this specific part of our chat and a common belief that can ironically result in dwindling motivation levels—the thought that you have to eat back the calories you burn.

Eating Back Calories Burnt

During my final year at university in Preston, I was deeply immersed in my Strength and Conditioning (S&C) degree, balancing internships at Preston North End FC and Wigan Warriors Rugby League Club, S&C coaching the university's female field hockey team, and enjoying life's simple pleasures, like 90s Dragon Ball reruns, the odd game of poker and meals out with friends.

Despite the chaos, I diligently tracked my food, aiming to maintain my weight by matching my calorie intake with the calorie burn reported by my smartwatch. Trusting the device's accuracy, I followed this plan for 3 months, only to find that I was gaining a considerable amount of weight, not maintaining it.

This unexpected outcome was a pivotal lesson about fitness trackers' reliability and calorie burn estimates. *It was a moment of realisation that these gadgets can significantly overestimate the calories burned.*

With those lessons learned and the education gained since, I want to emphasise a few things.

As mentioned, you shouldn't exercise merely to burn calories—you're not a hamster. It's crucial to understand that approaching exercise with a calorie-centric mindset can lead to an unhealthy relationship with physical activity. This inevitably leads to viewing exercise as a chore or punishment rather than the source of enjoyment and stress relief that it is.

Moreover, exercising merely to offset calorie intake removes your attention from where you should focus—like progressive overload. This is because you then do exercises that don't contribute to progress, hoping to burn as many calories as possible, such as burpees, sprinting on the spot and aimlessly jumping up and down. It's also important to mention again that a 30-minute workout makes up 2% of your day, and the real key to fat loss lies in what you do during the remaining 98% of your time.

Nowadays, I advise you to:

1. Approach the calorie burn feature within fitness trackers with a healthy dose of scepticism. Removing this feature, if possible, from your display is often more beneficial—which is precisely what I do.
2. Turn off the feature that your calorie tracking app may have, which adds the calories you've burnt throughout the day to your daily calorie goal.

Next up: the myth of spot reduction.

The Myth of "Spot Reduction"

As we continue our discussion on strength training, we must address a common misconception: the spot reduction myth.

What exactly is spot reduction? It's the belief that you can target fat loss in specific areas of your body by doing exercises focusing on them. For instance, the idea that performing abdominal exercises like planks or bicycle crunches will specifically reduce abdominal fat or that tricep exercises such as dips or cable extensions will burn fat off your triceps.

Unfortunately, this is a myth. Fat loss doesn't work selectively. You cannot choose where on your body to lose fat. It's similar to trying to empty only a specific corner of a swimming pool while hoping the rest remains level; in reality, when you remove water, the entire pool's level gradually lowers. This may be frustrating, especially when dealing with 'stubborn areas'— commonly the abdominal area for men and the glutes and thighs for women—but it is what it is.

So, what should you do if you aim to lose fat in a specific area? The solution is overall body fat reduction through a calorie deficit. Genetics and gender then typically determine where you lose fat "fastest" and "slowest" (for lack of a better term). For instance, I tend to lose fat from my face and thighs relatively quickly, while my lower back, chest, and abdominal areas are more resistant and take much longer. On the other hand, I have a friend who quickly gains fat on his face, yet his chest will lean down rapidly.

This doesn't mean it's impossible to lose fat from these stubborn areas; it just requires a longer period in a calorie deficit and potentially pushing yourself even further beyond your comfort zone. Just as the level of the entire pool lowers gradually as you continue to remove water, so too will these stubborn areas eventually respond to sustained efforts.

With that said, let's open up on you following your very own strength training routine.

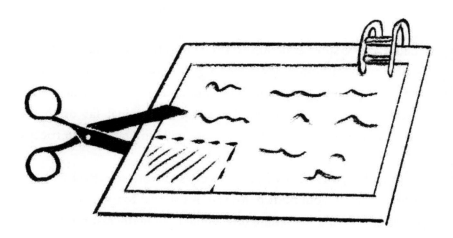

Chapter 6:
Starting Your
Strength Training Routine

One thing that I love more than a cup of coffee is a fantastic strength training session. Now, I understand that not everyone loves exercise. You might even hate it—but it's still got to get done. And truth be told, there are days when I can't be bothered to get it done either. However, I don't want to discuss strength training and exercise without educating you on how you can approach your routine.

So, let's get stuck in, starting with a common subject—gym intimidation.

Gym Intimidation

First, if you regularly workout at home, this section isn't for you. However, this could be perfect if you've been on the fence about joining a gym.

With that said, what's one question I get asked repeatedly?

No, it's not about who my favourite Peaky Blinders character is, my favourite convenience store snack in Japan, or why I accidentally ran into a closed door with full force back in secondary school.

It's actually, "Leo, how do I get over my gym intimidation?"

Chances are, you also probably think you're in the minority—but ironically, you're in the majority. Trust me when I say that many people have the same fears and anxieties as you regarding being scared to go to the gym. There's no "off/on switch" for gym intimidation either but doing your best to implement some of the following suggestions will help—and this is me speaking from experience.

First, let's get something straight: people at the gym are too wrapped up in their workouts to bother about what you're doing. Not the super-fit person bench pressing a small car or the one breezing through a challenging workout like it's nothing.

"But Leo, I feel like they are judging me."

Let's consider 2 possibilities:

Scenario 1: Maybe someone did look your way. But letting that worry stop you from hitting your fitness goals isn't the way to go. Should someone else's thoughts steer your life? Absolutely not. And if someone is judging, that's their problem, not yours. They might be dealing with their own issues and, unfortunately, projecting that onto others.

Scenario 2: Perhaps you're naturally feeling a tad self-conscious in a new environment and think someone's watching you. Most gym-goers are too focused on their routine to pay attention to anyone else for more than a few seconds. They might have glanced because they liked your outfit or were daydreaming between sets.

Now that we've tackled those worries, let's expand on practical steps to overcome gym intimidation.

- **Go in with a Plan:** A workout plan provides direction and reduces anxiety and the feeling of being watched by outlining exercises, sets, reps, and rest times. It ensures you're more confident of your next move and boosts confidence with clear goals and focus for each session.

- **The testosterzone:** If the dumbbell area, or 'testosterzone' as I've informally nicknamed it, feels intimidating, opt for machine-based exercises like chest or leg presses to still achieve an effective workout without entering the more daunting parts of the gym. For example, whenever I have a new 1-2-1 online fitness member who is self-conscious about stepping into this area, I'll program their first few workouts for the other parts of their gym.

- **Gradual Exposure:** Gradually acclimate to the gym using almost what's called exposure therapy. Start with a tour, progress to comfortable areas, consider classes, bring a friend, or work with a trainer to build familiarity and confidence.

- **Proper Preparation is Key:** Learn each exercise in your plan beforehand to avoid confusion. Dedicate time to familiarising yourself with the movements, which will help with safety and effectiveness while working out.

- **Accountability:** Seek external support by joining online or in-person fitness communities, hiring a personal trainer, or starting with online coaching. This support network can provide guidance, reduce the feeling of isolation, and increase your confidence. In fact, I rate seeking accountability so highly that I'll be expanding on it more later.

- **Consistent Times:** When I was living in South London and attending my local gym in Norbury, I'd familiarised myself with so many of the gym members who went at similar times, it got to the point where the community and space felt like a second home. Visiting the gym at consistent times helps with comfort in the environment and the people, making it feel more welcoming and reducing intimidation as you recognise familiar faces and realise you're not alone in your fitness journey.

All that said, there comes a time when you just have to go. Because the only way to eventually get over your gym intimidation is to actually go to the gym. As long as you keep holding it off and never going, that feeling of intimidation will only grow—it won't just magically vanish one day.

It's kinda like never going in the water because you can't swim. Eventually, you've got to get into the water and learn to overcome the fear. Nothing will ever change the fact that you've got to push yourself to be uncomfortable.

Yes, I understand you're hesitant to go to the gym, but part of life consists of doing things you don't like—especially when they're good for you. Forever avoiding things you find uncomfortable means you will not grow. Taking that step towards going to the gym will be the most powerful thing you can do after we finish our chat.

Having covered ways of getting into the gym, let's transition to the warm-up and cool-down.

Warm-ups and Cool-Downs

Warm-ups are vital to your workout routine and help minimise injury risks. A good warm-up includes dynamic stretches, which are active movements that prepare your muscles and joints for the exercise ahead and should ideally take no more than 5 to 10 minutes. Following dynamic stretches, doing lighter weights for the exercises you plan to perform can further prime your body. For instance, if you aim to deadlift 100 kg for 6 reps, you might start with 50 kg for 4 reps and then 75 kg for 3 reps, progressively working up to your target weight.

On the other hand, cool-downs may hold less importance than sometimes believed. The notion that skipping a cool-down leads to increased muscle soreness also lacks scientific backing. However, focusing on your breathing and gently transitioning from the heightened fight-or-flight state of activity to rest may be beneficial. This doesn't need to be overcomplicated; simple relaxation or gentle stretching might suffice.

I and many other coaches I know have skipped the cool-down for years, and we've been fine, suggesting that extensive cool-down routines may not be as important as a thorough warm-up.

An Example Exercise Routine

In this section, I'll provide an example exercise routine designed for 2 full-body workouts per week. Each session is expected to last between 50 and 70 minutes, assuming you follow the suggested rest periods and don't spend the session on your phone. This routine assumes no medical conditions or injuries and is suitable for individuals at all levels, from beginners to advanced.

Full Body A				
Warm-up				
Exercise	**Reps/Timing**	**Sets**	**Rest Time**	**Mindful Notes**
Hip Flexor Stretch	30 seconds on each side	2	15 seconds	Mobility Exercise
Ankle Dorsiflexion Rocks	10 on each side	2	15 seconds	Mobility Exercise
Main Session				
Goblet Squats	6-8	3	2.5 minutes	Use a dumbbell or kettlebell
Single Leg Seated Leg Curl	8-10	3	1 minute and 30 seconds	Start with your non-dominant leg
Single Arm Dumbbell Bent Over Row	6-8	3	Superset*	Start with your non-dominant arm
Standing Dumbbell Shoulder Press	6-8	3	Superset*	
Lat Pulldown	8-10	3	1 minute and 30 seconds	
Plank	45 to 60 seconds	2	1 minute	

Full Body B				
Warm-up				
Exercise	**Reps/Timing**	**Sets**	**Rest Time**	**Mindful Notes**
Half-Kneeling T-Spine Opener	10 on each side	2	15 seconds	Mobility Exercise
Frog Pose	30 seconds	2	15 seconds	Mobility Exercise
Main Session				
Chin-up Variation	4-6	3	Superset*	Assisted if Necessary
Push-Up Variation	AMRAP**	3	Superset*	On your knees if necessary
Barbell Romanian Deadlift	6-8	3	2.5 minutes	
Single Leg Glute Bridges	10-12	3	1 minute and 30 seconds	Start with your non-dominant leg
Leg Press	10-12	3	1 minute and 30 seconds	
Pallof Press	10-12	2	1 minute	

*A 'superset' involves performing 2 different exercises consecutively with little, such as a minute, to no rest in between.

**'AMRAP' stands for 'As Many Reps As Possible.' For instance, when doing AMRAP push-ups, you continue until you can't perform any more reps while maintaining good form.

If you're considering adopting a twice-weekly workout regimen, feel free to use the sessions above as inspiration. Remember that these routines can be adjusted to meet your needs and preferences.

Other workout splits you could potentially follow are:

- Three times weekly: Upper, Lower, Full Body
- Four times weekly: Upper A, Lower A, Upper B, Lower B
- Five times weekly: Upper, Lower, Push, Pull, Legs

Alternatively, if you want a free workout plan that you can follow 2, 3, or even 4 times weekly, then you can grab the free workout plan from my website at kairos.online/pdf-guides

Now that we've covered the example routine, let's turn your attention to something vital for your progression: progressive overload.

Progressive Overload

To introduce the concept of progressive overload, let's briefly discuss the tale of Milo of Croton, a 6th-century B.C. Greek wrestler, as an example of ancient wisdom.

As the story goes, Milo began lifting and carrying a newborn calf every day. He continued this as the calf grew, and by the time it had become a full-sized bull, Milo had developed the strength to carry it with ease. This story illustrates how gradually increasing the load can lead to significant strength gains.

Just like Milo's gradual increase, progressive overload is about continuously challenging your body to adapt and grow. Let's break down exactly how you can do this in your workouts.

Progressive overload is the slow increase of stress (the good kind) placed on your body over time. It's you boosting the intensity of your workouts to force your body to adapt and grow stronger. If progress is something you're struggling to come by, it could be because you're not applying progressive overload effectively—and perhaps you've instead been focusing on indicators that don't matter, such as how much you do or don't sweat.

Let's break down the different methods of progressive overload:

- **Add More Weight**: If you're lifting 20kg for 10 reps on a dumbbell row and it feels manageable, then it's time to increase the weight, aiming for the next increment, such as 22.5kg. This additional weight challenges your muscles further.

- **Do More Reps**: Progress can also mean doing more repetitions. For example, you've applied progressive overload if you can do 3 chin-ups one week and 4 the next.

- **Improve Form**: While debatable, and perhaps not progressive overload per se, improving your form is another form of progression. For instance, if performing 5 reps of an 80kg barbell deadlift feels tough one week but easier the next, you've progressed.

- **Adding Tempos**: If you follow a 2.1.2 tempo in your barbell squat one week—taking 2 seconds to lower, pausing for one second at the bottom, and taking 2 seconds to rise—and the next week, you switch to a 3.2.3 tempo, intentionally slowing down each phase of the squat with the same amount of weight, you're progressively overloading.

- **Increase Timings**: Another effective way to progressively overload is to overcome previous timing, like holding a plank for 70 seconds, whereas before, you did 60.

The key takeaway is that you must ensure some form of progressive overload in your workouts to make lasting progress. Without it, your fitness journey will stagnate, which is likely not your goal—considering we're having this chat.

It's also important to understand that while you may make quick progress initially in strength training, progress will eventually slow down. Even adding an extra rep or 1.25kg is significant progress. There will also be times when you won't progress weekly; expecting to add 2.5kg every week to an exercise like a barbell bent over row would total 130kg in a year and 260kg in 2 years, which many lifters never even achieve throughout their entire career—let alone within 2 years. So, remember that there are many ways of applying progressive overload during your workouts.

Remember, applying progressive overload assumes that you maintain good form; trying to progressively overload with poor form can increase the risk of injury and should be avoided.

Now that we've discussed progression, let's talk about how you can track your progress effectively.

Tracking Progress

Take a trip back with me to my exchange year in Vermont again.

Amidst the excitement of trying my first corndog (not for me), attending thrilling ice hockey games, and exploring New England, I was still often hitting the gym. By that point, going to the gym had become part of my identity—I continued because I knew it was good for me, even though I wasn't entirely certain what I was doing.

However, there was a problem.

Despite recovering from a nagging shoulder injury and maintaining consistency at the university gym, my progress had stalled quickly. Looking back, I realise the key issue: I had no plan and didn't log my workouts.

I was improvising my workouts on the spot, had no record of which exercises were effective or where I was plateauing, and I was lifting varying weights each session because I was relying on memory. This lack of tracking undermined the principle of progressive overload.

A couple of years later, based on advice from an experienced gym-goer, I started logging my workouts—and saw my progress skyrocket.

It was then that I learned that the practice of logging your workouts is crucial for progression. Without tracking, you're essentially guessing your way through your workouts, which often leads to missed opportunities for growth. Like I said, logging your workouts also helps you realise which exercises are working best for you and which exercises you aren't progressing well with.

There are several effective methods I recommend for keeping track of your strength training progress, which have worked well for both me and my 1-2-1 online fitness members:

- **Digital Logging:** Use your smartphone or other handheld devices for a quick and convenient way to record your workouts, such as using your notes. However, I find this method also tends to be the most distracting.
- **Spreadsheets:** If you prefer a more organised and detailed approach, spreadsheets can be great.
- **Pen and Paper:** The classic method of writing things down always stays in style and is a reliable way to keep a physical record of your progress.

Some might say, "Leo, I can remember all my gym workouts." While that's great, it's doubtful you can recall every weight lifted for every rep and set, especially when life is filled with countless other details to remember.

I made this same mistake in Vermont.

Heck, I can't even remember what I had for lunch 2 days ago!

Anyway, let's look at how you might log your workouts. Suppose you're doing a dumbbell chest press for 3 sets of 8 to 10 reps, followed by a barbell overhead press. You could potentially log it like this:

- Dumbbell Chest Press
  - 25kg x 9 reps
  - 25kg x 8 reps
  - 25kg x 6 reps
- Barbell Overhead Press
  - 20kg x 10 reps
  - 20kg x 10 reps
  - 20kg x 8 reps

Here, the first number is the weight lifted, followed by the number of reps listed for each set.

Remember, logging your workouts isn't a do-or-die requirement but a tool that can catapult your progress. It only takes a few seconds between sets, and when you're resting, sometimes up to 4 minutes, that's plenty of time to do it.

I log my workouts about 95% of the time. I might skip it for a vacation workout or a session at a new gym, but for the most part, it's a part of my routine.

Now that we've covered that, let's move forward with a bit on muscle soreness.

Muscle Soreness or DOMS (Delayed Onset Muscle Soreness)

Chilling on my grandad's favourite chair in his South London home, as I watched football on Portuguese cable television, I spotted an old 5kg dumbbell lying around, gathering dust for years. On a whim, I decided to give it a go, performing the only exercise I knew: bicep curls.

Positioned right in front of the T.V., I mindlessly curled that dumbbell, doing well over a hundred reps per arm—possibly even double or triple that. It was my first-ever attempt at weight training, and I went at it without any notion of structure, rest, good form, or variety.

The following day brought a shock.

My arms were in such intense, unfamiliar soreness that even basic movements felt impossible. I remember standing helplessly in the supermarket with my dad, unable to extend my arm to grab orange juice off the top shelf when he asked me to.

This experience is me saying that you shouldn't be going as hard as possible when first starting with your workouts. The first few weeks should be you laying the foundation, such as:

- Getting comfortable at the gym
- Learning movement patterns, e.g. deadlifts, squats and overhead presses
- Getting to know your body

Very intense soreness isn't a badge of success; it often means you did too much. Progress isn't about soreness but about improving over time, like lifting heavier weights or mastering form. Although saying that, never having any soreness at all might mean your workouts likely need more intensity. So, as you can see, just like many things, there's a middle ground.

To recover from soreness, focus on quality protein intake, rest days, and minimising alcohol intake.

Having discussed everyday movement, NEAT, and strength training, let's move on to a topic that perfectly complements these: the importance of recovery in your fitness journey.

Chapter 7:
The Critical Role of
Rest and Recovery

The importance of recovery has been recognised throughout history and across cultures, each with its traditions and practices emphasising the need for rest.

With that said, let's move away from the reality of our coffee shop setting and, for a second, imagine yourself at the restorative Roman Baths to the tranquil Japanese Onsens, or even move to ancient China, in which they'd share the philosophy of balancing Yin (rest) and Yang (activity). What you'd see is that for thousands of years, many societies have long known that progress and self-improvement are as much about the periods of rest as they are about the times of activity.

So when it comes to rest in fitness or life in general, why do some people think they're above it?

This section expands on the role recovery plays in fitness and human health.

Rest Days

When you strength train, you're making tiny muscle tears. Don't worry; this is good because when you rest, your body fixes those, and your muscles grow back stronger. Resting also helps reduce physical fatigue, leaving you feeling more energised for future workouts and less prone to injury. However, if you don't take rest days and keep working out, your body doesn't have the chance to fix those tears. It's like if you got a small cut on your finger and kept picking at it instead of letting it heal.

Now, in my coaching experience, chances are, you fall into one of 2 categories regarding rest days:

- **The Rest Day Ignorers:** You fear taking rest days and worry that pausing equals regression. You believe that without constant activity, progress will slip away.
- **The Inconsistent Gym-goer:** On the flip side, you may only follow a workout routine sporadically. Naturally, this results in excessive rest days. If this is you, you might not need to prioritise this "rest days" section as much, but it's still beneficial to understand the value of structured rest.

On my own rest days, I allocate the time I'd usually spend commuting and training to other important activities—communicating with my 1-2-1 online fitness members, managing household chores, tending to the plants, organising my schedule, and studying. However, rest days don't mean complete inactivity; I stay active with tasks that keep me moving throughout the day and might also engage in low-intensity activities like going for a stroll or meeting friends for a coffee.

Anyway, I can see why this happens regarding the "more is always better" fitness mindset. It's a concept that often holds in many aspects of life:

- More studies of physics lead to a more knowledgeable person in physics.
- More French language practice results in greater fluency in French.

- More hours practising piano creates a more skilled musician.
- More time spent painting improves artistic skill and expression.
- More driving leads to more experience behind the wheel.

However, regarding physical training and our bodies, this principle of 'more' isn't necessarily the case. *It must be balanced with adequate rest.* For example, in fitness:

- More strength training can potentially lead to overuse injuries, such as tennis elbow.
- More intensity without rest periods can potentially lead to diminished returns and plateaus.
- More running miles might lead to injuries like shin splints or stress fractures.

However, like I said, 'more' can sometimes be better, especially if you've been largely inconsistent. For example, if you've been off-track with your nutrition and workouts, increasing your commitment will benefit you. So, unlike what some bubbles of social media today may have people believe, a middle ground can and does exist.

When it comes to determining the ideal number of rest days, various factors will influence your decision, including your training experience, specific fitness goals, workout intensity, available time, and the nature of your exercise routine. However, if you're following a strength training program that focuses on progressive overload, I generally recommend *at least* 2 rest days per week for recovery and muscle repair.

Now, let's move on from rest days to rest times, which are the breaks you take between sets during a workout.

Rest Times

One warm autumn evening back when I lived in Osaka, after enjoying a delicious bento box from the local convenience store, a day exploring Ebisubashi Bridge and trying takoyaki for the first time, I got a text from Adam. Adam, a 1-2-1 online fitness member, a great friend from South London, and an avid e-gamer who works in IT support, was a few months into consistently working out for the first time.

His message read, "Leo, is it okay if I rest for less time between my sets of deadlifts?" He quickly added, "Because I don't feel the need to rest as long between sets."

I had initially suggested about two and a half minutes of rest, give or take thirty seconds, but I was intrigued by his messages. They hinted that Adam might not be pushing himself enough during his deadlifts. Typically, if you're lifting a challenging enough weight, you'd cherish every second of rest, maybe even wishing for a bit more.

So, I asked him to send a video of him doing the deadlift. Sure enough, he wasn't pushing himself anywhere near as much as he could. My advice was simple: "No, increase the weight instead. Your form is great, but the video shows you're stronger than you think."

Adam's follow-up message made me smile the next week: "Leo, is it okay if I rest a little longer? LOL"

This story about Adam illustrates an essential point regarding your rest periods dictating whether or not you're strength training. For example, if you rest for 20 seconds in between sets, even if you're using weights, you're not strength training.

I often see another common error regarding rest times between sets: not actually resting. For example, if your idea of resting between sets involves burpees, push-ups, or running on the spot, let's be clear—you're not resting.

So, what should you be doing instead? Well, rest.

Sit, stand, stroll—whatever allows you to recover without tiring yourself further. This break is crucial for preparing your body for the next set.

How long should you rest? It's tough to give specifics without knowing more context, but for isolation exercises, you'd do well to rest for about a minute to 2 minutes. For compound exercises, resting anywhere from 2 to 4 minutes if you've just completed a strenuous set can work–similar to what Adam consistently aimed for after.

In summary, take your rest times seriously by actually resting. If your training program's recommended rest periods seem too long, it's a strong indicator that you might need to increase your lift's intensity, perhaps by adding more weight or doing more reps.

With that said, let's move on to another form of rest—sleep.

Sleep's Relationship with Weight Management

Have you ever wondered why fat loss still seems like an uphill battle despite hitting the gym regularly and eating well? One reason could be your sleep. Sleep isn't just a "big block of nothingness", and it goes way beyond simply dreaming about laying on a beach in Cuba or your club winning European football cups (as a Crystal Palace fan, I can certainly dream)—sleep is essential for fat loss and life. Everything feels infinitely harder when you're sleep-deprived.

Sleep deserves massive respect. Unfortunately, many people aren't giving it that.

First, consider how a fluctuating weekend schedule that causes you to stay up late can disrupt your sleep, much like a mild case of jet lag. On Friday and Saturday nights, many people stay up late and then sleep in the next morning. This messes with your body's natural sleep schedule—similar to how you feel when you travel across time zones. By Sunday, your sleep pattern is out of sync, making Monday and Tuesday tough as you try to get back on track. You might feel groggy and tired as you struggle to catch up on sleep. Although you might recover by Wednesday, the cycle starts all over again each weekend, trapping you in a constant loop of sleep disruption.

Then, remember what I said in the water and hydration section about chronic dehydration becoming a person's new norm in which they'll eventually no longer be able to distinguish the difference? I feel the same way about sleep. Many people live in a state of chronic sleep deprivation without even realising it. This chronic sleep deprivation might happen for so long that it subtly establishes itself as your 'new normal'. The tell-tale signs of feeling overly tired become something you're used to. As a result, you might think you're someone who can function perfectly fine on less sleep. However, it's actually that you've just been accustomed to feeling overly tired for way too long. I've seen this happen firsthand with close friends.

More sleep would do you the world of good (RIP new parents).

Now, there are various reasons why fat loss feels much more challenging when coupled with sleep deprivation—one of which is also due to its impact on hunger hormones like ghrelin and leptin.

Ghrelin is like an "encourager", nudging you towards another slice of pizza. At the same time, leptin is the voice that signals when you've had enough. A good balance of both is necessary, but when sleep deprivation enters the picture, ghrelin gets louder, and leptin fades into the background. This imbalance can lead to excessive snacking and late-night kitchen raids, often not for the healthiest options.

So, how can you enhance your sleep quality? Here are some strategies to consider, in no particular order:

- Begin winding down an hour or 2 before bedtime.
- Opt for calming sounds and avoid stimulating sounds, songs or movies.
- Avoid alcohol and heavy meals close to bedtime.
- Use your device's night shift and filter settings to reduce blue light exposure.
- Engage in screen-free, relaxing activities like reading, drawing, meditating, gentle stretching, or puzzles. This one works especially well when you consider that social media apps we often use frequently push emotionally charged or controversial content to keep users engaged. Rather than helping you relax, this can leave you feeling amped up or annoyed.
- Keep a consistent sleep schedule, waking up and going to bed at the same times daily to regulate your internal clock.
- Minimise or even eliminate caffeine about 8 hours before bedtime.

This isn't to say you have to follow all the above suggestions. However, implementing at least a couple of these and prioritising 7 to 8 hours of quality sleep most nights will only help.

Caffeine

You may be wondering why on Earth I've mentioned caffeine right after the sleep section of our chat, considering it's known to keep you up and ready for the hustle and bustle of the day ahead. However, that's precisely why I'm mentioning it—because it's the most commonly abused drug in today's society, and many people, potentially yourself included, don't realise how caffeine negatively impacts your sleep.

I also know it's ironic that we're chatting about caffeine's potential adverse effects while we're at a coffee shop enjoying our own cups but consider this: if caffeine chronically disrupts your sleep, it will inevitably hinder your progress in fat loss.

While it's true that a segment of the population are non-responders to caffeine—like my dad, who can down a cup of coffee and sleep like a rock—most people likely overestimate their immunity to its effects. Instead, I believe many people have grown accustomed to a baseline of sleep deprivation and poor sleep, using caffeine as a crutch to counteract tiredness, not realising it perpetuates a cycle of disrupted sleep and further reliance on caffeine.

For example, having lived in Portugal, where my parents are from, I've been immersed in an espresso-loving culture. A typical day in Portugal for the locals, including my friends and family, might go:

Breakfast. Double Espresso. Lunch. Espresso. Snack. Espresso. Dinner. Espresso.

The post-dinner espresso will often be around 9 to 10p.m., a common practice despite the late hour.

This habitual intake, embraced culturally, reminds us that sometimes we may be unaware of excessive habits, as it could be the norm we've grown up with. This personal reflection isn't just about caffeine either—it's also about understanding the broader implications of our daily routines on sleep and health.

If you're a coffee lover like me, you'll be glad to hear I'm not here to tell you to stop drinking coffee. Instead, to break this cycle, try simple adjustments like going to bed a bit earlier or avoiding caffeine after 3p.m. The solution might seem too straightforward, but the simplest answers are often the most effective.

Now, let's explore the next chapter, which massively impacts fat loss and your life as a whole.

Chapter 8:
The Power of Mindset in Fat Loss Success

As I lean in from my plush chair during this coffee shop chat, it's time to tell you about perhaps the most pivotal part of any fitness journey—your psychology.

This part of our chat will cover the power of mindset, belief systems, and common hurdles like fear of failure, past traumas, and societal pressures, equipping you with a few practical strategies to overcome these obstacles. Plus, from all my years of coaching people, it's clear that where you're at mentally is one of the most significant indicators of sustainable health and fitness progress—and ironically, it's a subject that often gets pushed to the backseat of fat loss journeys.

Often, it's not just about the food or the workouts; it's about what's going on upstairs—in your mind. Beliefs, attitudes, and mindsets can either catapult us forward or hold us back. Your self-efficacy, otherwise known as your belief in your ability to handle situations or achieve goals, will be the ultimate dictator for whether or not you succeed.

Anyway, let's get stuck in.

Disclaimer:
The insights shared in this chapter regarding the psychology of fat loss are based on my experiences, academic background in select psychology

modules, and observations from coaching people worldwide. I am not a licensed psychologist or mental health professional.

- While many have found the following tips and insights beneficial, they are general suggestions that may not apply to you.
- If you find yourself grappling with psychological or emotional concerns, please seek advice and guidance from a licensed mental health professional, not this book.
- The mental and emotional aspects of fat loss are complex and individualised. This chapter aims to provide a broad understanding and helpful tools. It is not absolute nor a substitute for professional advice.

Understanding Mindsets: The Difference Between Fixed and Growth

Looking up the definition of mindset, you'll find it means "the established set of attitudes held by someone."

Therefore, let's chat about something I learned before becoming a coach. It was introduced to me briefly at school and then on a deeper level at sixth form and university, and it has stuck with me since.

The 2 types of mindsets: fixed and growth.

Imagine you're playing a card game. Having a fixed mindset is kinda like getting a poor hand of cards and thinking, "Well, this is the hand I've been dealt. Guess I'm stuck with it. This game is not going to go well." But someone with a growth mindset? They believe they can still play a good game with a solid strategy, even if dealt a lousy hand. Those with a growth mindset tackle challenges head-on, bounce back from setbacks, and are generally more successful. Gradually adopting a growth mindset can be like a secret weapon in fat loss, where the journey has many ups and downs.

Of course, a growth mindset doesn't fix everything, but it can certainly play a massive part in anyone's success.

Sometimes, it's easy to read about something negative, e.g., fixed mindsets, and then to quickly get defensive and claim, "That's not me". However, if you're the type of person who sees people you know have success with their fat loss, and rather than thinking, "If they can do it, I can do it too" or "Wow, maybe they'll be a great resource or have some great tips for me", and instead, you'll justify it with why they achieved it, and why you haven't, e.g. they have more money, time etc. You may have more of a fixed mindset than you realise.

This isn't being said to take digs at you—remember, everything I'm sharing with you here is from a place of love and a genuine desire to see you improve. So, it's crucial to realise instances where a fixed mindset might be at play and do your best to gradually progress towards a growth mindset.

However, I get it; it's *way easier said than done.*

So, let's make it actionable.

Here are a few practical tips to get your mindset moving in the direction of being more "growth mindset" oriented for your fat loss journey:

1. Embrace the Power of "Yet".
Whenever you think, "I can't do this," add a magical word at the end: "yet." Suddenly, "I can't do this" transforms into "I can't do this yet." This simple word change creates a powerful feeling of potential.

2. Visualise Your Success.
Spend time imagining your daily fat loss journey as a series of successful steps. Picture yourself overcoming challenges and reaching your goals. Visualisation can boost your confidence and motivation.

3. Positive Affirmations.

Create and repeat positive affirmations that resonate with your goals. For example, "I am strong and capable. I make healthy choices every day." Affirmations can help rewire your thought patterns.

4. Set Achievable Milestones.

Break your fat loss journey into smaller, achievable milestones. Rather than telling yourself you need to lose 15kg, focus on being 85% consistent with training, steps and protein goals for the next 3 months, then review it afterwards. Celebrate your successes along the way. These victories reinforce your growth mindset and keep you motivated.

5. Be Your Best Friend.

Imagine you said everything you say about yourself to your best friend. Would you tell your friends that they can't do it and will never succeed? Obviously not. So, why say those things to yourself? A growth mindset means being your supportive and encouraging friend on this journey.

We can even take it further and see some of the above examples applied.

- "I've tried before, and it was a flop. Fat loss isn't for me."
  - Embracing the Power of Yet: "Every stumble is a martial arts move I haven't figured out yet. Each attempt gets me closer to my goal."
- "Man, fat loss feels like playing a football game in which the other team has all the star players!"
  - Positive Affirmation: "Challenges just make the story better. With the right strategy and persistence, I will win this."
- "Ugh, willpower and I broke up ages ago."
  - Being Your Best Friend: "I went through a lot previously. I'm at a different point in my life now. I'm ready to crush this journey!"

The Astonishing Power of the Placebo Effect

Now that you've understood fixed and growth mindsets, let's talk about one of the most powerful and under-discussed aspects of psychology, something that'll play a massive role in your health and fitness journey: the placebo and nocebo effects.

The Placebo Effect: Your Mind's Magic Trick

The placebo effect isn't just about feeling better after taking a sugar pill, thinking it's medicine; it's about genuine physical changes and progression that can occur simply because you believe they will. Even the higher cost of something can be a placebo, in which you'll think it to be of higher value, better effectiveness, or even more likely to be more consistent with it.

The placebo effect is so strong that it must be accounted for in scientific research.

A personal favourite example of the placebo effects power on display is sham surgeries. Patients go through all the motions of surgery—the preparation, anaesthesia, and the incision—but no actual surgical procedure is performed.

However, this is where it gets interesting—because many patients still report relief from their symptoms, all because their minds were convinced that a surgery had just happened!

This effect extends beyond medicine and into the world of sport, too. Research on the placebo effect indicates that athletes' beliefs about the effectiveness of an intervention significantly affect their performance. For instance, athletes run faster when they believe they've ingested caffeine or think a placebo will enhance performance.

Now, consider how this applies to your fat loss and fitness journey. Imagine having this power of belief in your daily routine. When you start your morning workout or choose a healthier meal option, believe in the positive impact of that choice on your body. Tell yourself, "This workout is making me stronger," or "Eating this healthy meal is nourishing my body"—it can be as simple as that.

Of course, I understand that if you're "aware of a placebo", then it's not a placebo—but interestingly, the placebo effect can still occur even when you know it's at play. The 'open-label placebo' shows that the process and your belief are still powerful, highlighting how context and mindset are just as important as the action.

Now, as we explore the power of belief through the placebo effect, remember that this power can work in both positive and negative ways. This brings us to its counterpart—the nocebo effect.

The Nocebo Effect: Mind Over Matter in Reverse

The nocebo effect is the placebo effect's less talked about sibling, but just as powerful.

Imagine this: you're trying a new health routine, but deep down, you're convinced it won't work. *This belief alone can set you up for a self-fulfilling prophecy of failure.*

The nocebo effect occurs when negative expectations lead to adverse outcomes. It's a psychological boomerang. What you send out regarding negative thoughts comes back to you as unfavourable results. These expectations end up physically manifesting in your body.

For instance, constantly thinking, "This new eating approach is going to be another letdown," or "I'll never get fit," can inhibit your progress. For example, your body might respond to these negative beliefs by lowering your energy levels, making workouts feel harder, or even affecting how often you decide to be consistent, e.g. skipping another day at the gym or saying yes to the fourth treat that day because "you'll never achieve your fitness goal anyway."

Recognising the nocebo effect at play is the first step in combating it. When you catch yourself slipping into negative thought patterns, pause momentarily. Challenge those thoughts. Ask yourself, "Are these beliefs based on facts, or are they just inner fears speaking?"

Acknowledging and transforming negative thought processes isn't about ignoring reality but reframing your perspective. It's about shifting from "I can't do this" to "I'm learning how to do this." Recognising that every step, even the small and uncertain ones, is part of becoming a healthier you. It's about actively improving your chances of success.

Before moving on to the next section, I want you to pause and reflect on your fitness journey. Have there been moments when your belief in a diet's effectiveness made it work better for you? Or a time when you doubted a workout regimen so much that it failed before you even gave it a fair chance.

These instances are not mere coincidences but the placebo and nocebo effects at play in your life.

So, as we sip our coffee and ponder, consider the potential of your own beliefs.

The Physiological Impact of Mindset

While mindset influences actions and behaviours, it also has physiological effects.

A positive and growth-oriented mindset can promote stress reduction, leading to a more balanced hormonal environment in the body. It also promotes overall well-being and can boost the body's immunity and metabolic processes, indirectly influencing fat loss outcomes. Whereas chronic stress, for instance, can elevate cortisol levels, which is linked to increased belly fat.

To illustrate this further, let's consider the example of 2 guys starting a fat loss journey.

Person A, who we'll call Bob, approaches his fat loss journey with a positive and growth-oriented mindset. Bob believes in his ability to make positive changes and views challenges as opportunities to learn and grow.

Person B, on the other hand, Bill, has a negative and fixed mindset. Bill doubts his ability to succeed, often feels overwhelmed by challenges, and views setbacks as failures.

Now, let's look at the physiological effects over time.

Bob's positive mindset reduces stress levels, making it easier to fall asleep, stay asleep, and gather the energy to get up and go to the gym. Lower stress levels also mean less cortisol, a hormone associated with fat storage. Bob's immune system functions more efficiently; inside, he's in a better balance. All of these factors indirectly contribute to his success in fat loss.

In contrast, Bill's negative mindset keeps him under constant stress. Elevated cortisol levels make it harder for him to fall asleep and shed those extra pounds. He often feels tired and run down; his ghrelin (the hunger hormone) is then higher. Overall, he finds it challenging to stay active and motivated. The negative mindset is like an anchor holding him back from his fat loss goals.

So, in the grand scheme of things? The mind's got a massive say in your fat loss journey. Both directly, in your daily choices and behaviours, and indirectly, through physiological responses.

Working towards adopting a growth-focused mindset can be the game-changer you've been looking for. Because remember, fat loss is as much about what's in your mind as it is about food and workouts. Embrace setbacks as learning opportunities, challenge negative thoughts, and stay kind to yourself.

Each small step forward counts.

Chapter 9:
Overcoming Mental Barriers to Fat Loss

Now that we've explored the power of a growth-oriented mindset, picture our cups steaming gently as we sit face-to-face in the coffee shop as I tell you about the mental roadblocks hindering your fat loss journey. This will be followed by an example of how it hinders it and then a friendly reminder for you to note down.

1) Fear of Failure: Have you ever started something thinking, "What if I can't do it?" We've all been there. It's like wanting to dive into a pool but not doing it because you fear the cold water even before you touch it.

Reframe Failure: You know when you try a new recipe, and it doesn't turn out exactly how you expected? You didn't 'fail' at cooking; you just learned what to adjust for next time. Look at setbacks the same way. Each stumble is a lesson, not a failure.

2) Past Traumas: Past events, like the mean comments you never forgot from Physical Education (P.E.) class at school that dented your confidence.

Talk it Out: Similar to how you may vent about your week, sometimes it helps to chat about those past hurts. Talking can be therapeutic, whether with a close buddy or a professional.

3) Societal Pressures: Have you ever felt the weight of all those 'perfect' images on digital platforms?

Limit Exposure: In a world of photoshoots and social media models, it can be easy to fall into the trap of spending your entire life restricting food. Exhausting, right? Maybe take a break from or limit time on digital platforms, or even think twice about who you follow and subscribe to. Focus on your journey, rather than focusing on trainers who profit off glamourising unrealistically low levels of body fat but don't like to mention the awful quality of life that comes with it.

4) Comparing to Others: Imagine seeing someone with the same goal as yours but seemingly achieving it effortlessly. That hint of envy you feel? Note it.

Real vs. Ideal: Remember that many images are curated, edited, or posed. Real life is more messy and less perfect. You're comparing your regular to someone else's miniature highlight reel.

5) Low Self-Worth: Have you ever felt like no matter what achievements you gain, they're never good enough? That's how low self-worth manifests.

Highlight Success: Start keeping a journal or a list of your achievements, no matter how small. For example, that day you chose a salad over chips for the first time or did one more push-up than last week. Recognise your wins. I'll share a great example of this with you from my 1-2-1 online fitness member, Melissa, soon.

6) Fear of Success: Worrying about people treating you differently once you progress.

Embrace Change: Gaining experience and changing as the years go by is precisely what life is about.

7) Setting Unrealistic Expectations: It's like expecting a flower to bloom immediately after planting its seed. Progress takes time.

Reality Check: Let's aim for things that are a stretch but still doable. If we expect to climb Everest overnight, maybe it's time to start with a hill first.

Unpacking these barriers can feel a little heavy at times, but shining a light on them is the first step to understanding and becoming the best version of yourself. Your health and fitness journey goes beyond physical changes because mental matters, too, and the more you train the mental side, the stronger it becomes—just like a muscle.

Plus, you don't have to face these barriers alone, either. Surround yourself with a supportive community, whether friends, family, a support group, or even online communities filled with people walking a similar path.

If any of these barriers ring a bell, know you're not alone. Regardless of changing trends, folks like you and I have always faced these challenges in every corner of the world. Isn't knowing that others have felt like you throughout history comforting? It's like we're all in a massive tapestry of humanity that's been woven together.

Remember: the mind and body are intrinsically linked. What you've learned here lays the foundation for everything else we've been discussing and will continue to.

Next up, and going beyond physical changes, we're diving into "deepening your motivation." Trust me, you won't want to miss this.

Deepening Your Motivation

Earlier in our chat, we explored workout motivation, emphasising the sequence of Action → Results → Motivation. Now, let's understand your 'why' for fat loss. It may sound cliché, but understanding, writing, and frequently revisiting your core motivation can only help.

Consider this dialogue as an example of digging deeper into your 'why':

- You: "I want to look better."
- Me: "Why?"
- You: "I want more confidence."
- Me: "Why is that confidence important?"
- You: "When I was younger, I felt more confident and miss that feeling."
- Me: "Miss that feeling?"
- You: "I want to regain confidence because I feel a change in how all my once favourite clothes now fit, and it hurts."

As this conversation continues, we uncover layers beneath the initial goal of 'looking better.' It's about regaining confidence, rekindling connections, ensuring family stability, and reigniting self-assurance in your career. This depth in your 'why' is what will catapult you forward on days when motivation seems low. While this specific example might not apply to you, diving deeper into your reasons could uncover a powerful driving force.

On the note of motivation throughout your fitness journey, this also brings up perhaps one of the most valuable tips I've encountered throughout my career from my 1-2-1 online fitness member, Melissa—who I briefly introduced near the beginning of this whole chat.

One day, out of the blue, she messaged me, word for word, with the following:

"Just wanted to share a list I've been keeping since working with you, and I'm loving the fact that I still haven't stopped adding stuff to it! Every time I have a positive thought about my journey so far, I add it here. And it's been great!"

Here's her list of compiled wins that she preceded to share with me:

- I've gone two sizes down on my smart watch around my wrist
- My belly bar now sits straight and not slanted
- I can put my socks on without holding my breath
- I can stand in front of the mirror
- My favourite jumper is now too baggy
- I ordered a replacement jumper, size S
- I have better stamina
- Fell in love with cycling again
- Confident enough to show my latest tattoo
- I am not afraid to stay on track, and I openly tell people I calorie count without feeling like I have to lie
- When did I begin to obsess over walking?
- Tying shoelaces is super easy now, too
- I can touch my toes with my legs straight
- The scale is my friend
- It's okay to have Biscoff Latte more than once a week
- Untracked meals are my friend
- I've had to replace my bras twice so far as they're too big
- I can walk for ages, and my knees and feet are fine

- I've gone down from a size 20 to a 14; my bank account does not appreciate it
- I've had to redo my Face ID on my phone as my face is slimming down, and it works less and less each time.

I had no idea she had composed this list of her wins as we worked together. Still, I'm glad she had done so, as it only added to her motivation on more challenging days. I immediately became a fan of writing down and listing your wins, no matter how small you may deem them to be.

So, perhaps take inspiration from my 1-2-1 online fitness member and good friend, Melissa, and try it yourself.

Next up: the comparison trap.

The Comparison Trap

Do the following scenarios sound familiar?

Scenario A: Misjudging Others' Eating Habits

You notice Declan from work indulging in a couple of doughnuts and half a pizza without care while you're battling frustration because it seems like he can eat anything and still lose weight.

Meanwhile, you feel just one takeaway meal throws you back to square one, especially when you notice a significant spike in your scale weight the next day.

We'll expand on the fact that scale weight fluctuations are massively influenced by many factors beyond just fat loss or gain later, so I'll save that conversation for now. Instead, what's crucial to address here is the danger of falling into the comparison trap. Observing someone else's eating and feeling disheartened because it appears they're progressing and you're not is pointless. The truth is, you don't know what Declan—or anyone else for that matter—is eating or doing 98% of the time.

Declan may have been super consistent with his diet over the past few weeks, crushed his workouts for the last 6 months, and had 90% consistency with his daily 20-minute walks for a year—and the moment you're seeing is just that—a moment where he's chosen to indulge a bit more than usual.

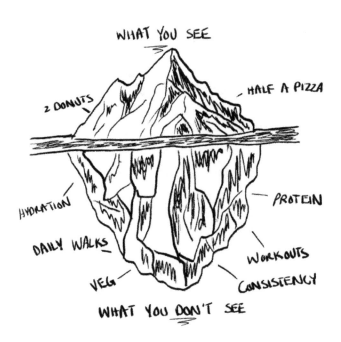

Scenario B: Beware of Quick Fix Diets

Watching Mai, a family friend, quickly lose weight on the keto diet might make you doubt your approach and feel frustrated about your "slower" progress. It might lead you to think, "Shall I ditch my plan and switch to keto?" or "Why am I not getting results like she is?"

But it's crucial to remember that rapid weight loss, like Mai's 5kg drop in a couple of weeks, is often water weight, especially at the beginning of such diets. Also, consider that this is Mai's eighth diet in the last 18 months, and she's regained the lost weight each time due to the unsustainability of her methods.

While your progress may seem slower, it's steady and sustainable, helping you avoid the exhausting cycle of yo-yo dieting. Slow and steady wins the race and ensures you don't have to keep running it repeatedly.

Scenario C: The Social Media Fitness Illusion

Genetics undoubtedly influence fitness progress by affecting appetite, muscle building capacity, recovery rates and more. Yet, a significant issue today is the constant comparison to individuals who represent the top 0.01% of fitness genetics.

Social media algorithms, aiming to maximise user engagement for profit, frequently showcase outrageous content—which includes these exceptional physiques, skewing your perception of "normal" and fuelling body dysmorphia.

To counter this, it's helpful to ground yourself in reality. Take a walk on any busy street worldwide, whether in Boston, Beijing or Brasília and observe the people around you. You'll notice that the extraordinary physiques seen online are not the norm. Constantly comparing yourself to the genetic elite—or others who aren't transparent about their use of performance-enhancing substances (which is more common than you might think!)—can harm your self-esteem and distort your view of your own progress.

My advice is to be highly aware of who you continuously watch, follow and subscribe to.

It is crucial to recognise and appreciate your unique fitness journey without measuring it against the rarest genetic outliers and deceptive images often seen online.

With these common scenarios outlined, you can see that comparison in all instances does nothing.

The reality is that regardless of the endeavour, there will always be someone you'll feel is doing better than you. You could build the tallest fucking skyscraper, only to see an even taller one pierce the horizon elsewhere.

I know it's cliché, but it's true—it's you versus you throughout this fitness thing. Recognising this can shift your perspective and help you avoid unhelpful comparisons.

With that covered, let's discuss the all-or-nothing mindset in fitness.

The All-or-Nothing Mindset

The 'all-or-nothing' mindset in fitness and fat loss is a perspective where your journey is seen in extremes: either you're fully committed, doing everything perfectly, or you're entirely off track, feeling like a failure. This way of thinking often leads to cycles of intense, unsustainable periods of exercise and strict dieting, followed by phases of inactivity and unhealthy eating.

Let's use an example.

Picture this: It's Friday night, and you're out with friends, enjoying pizza (ham and cheese on mine, please), a few beers, and even a pastel de nata (if you know, you know). As the evening wraps up and you're ready for bed, it hits you—you've gone massively over your calorie goal for the day, and the realisation is disheartening.

From here, you have 2 different mindset options:

Mindset A: "'I've messed up big time. I blew past my calorie limit and undid all the month's hard work. I might as well top it off with a whole bag of cookies since the day's already ruined, so there's no point.'

Mindset B: "So what? I had a great time with friends and created some wonderful memories, and yes, I went over my calorie count for a night. But it was worth it. I've been consistent for over 3 weeks and have made significant progress overall. Tomorrow, I'm back to being consistent—no biggie.'

Ask yourself, which mindset sounds like they will make long-term fitness progress?

The answer is clear.

Expecting setbacks is a realistic part of any fitness journey. They happen to everyone. Remember, it's never about the one "bad" day, week or even month—it's always about how you react to it. No one derails their fitness progress or gets out of shape from brief setbacks. An actual decline in health and fitness happens when you let these setbacks discourage you, leading to quitting and having prolonged poor habits. *Focus on maximising consistency rather than dwelling on temporary slip-ups.*

This nicely brings us to the myth of perfection.

The Myth of Perfection

Navigating a fitness journey is like exploring new territory; you can't expect to know everything from the start. For instance, consider if I aimed for perfection while learning Japanese, a language I initially knew nothing about. From day one, I'd quickly become overwhelmed and discouraged if I demanded flawless study sessions or mastery of all 3 Japanese alphabets—Hiragana, Katakana, and the daunting 2,136 Kanji characters.

So, just as learning a language reveals its depth and nuances over time, fitness unfolds new layers as you progress.

You can't ever be perfect with something you're only beginning to understand.

Striving for perfection in fitness and nutrition is unrealistic and unnecessary. Consistent efforts are far more effective than sporadic attempts at perfection—not just with fitness or language learning, but with everything in life. Labelling yourself as a 'perfectionist' and using it as an excuse to quit when things aren't perfect is a self-imposed limitation. *You're giving yourself a cop-out whenever the going inevitably gets tough.*

On the topic of toughness, let's now discuss common challenges.

Chapter 10:
Overcoming Common Challenges

This section will cover various fat loss challenges I've typically encountered as a coach. But before that, I want to tell you about my 1-2-1 online fitness member and friend, who's built a lovely life in Oslo—Laura.

She's a busy, dedicated professional who has tried almost every diet. Each attempt to lose weight felt like an uphill climb; she would make progress for a few weeks, only to slide back into old habits when stress and reality hit.

Laura's journey wasn't unlike Sisyphus's endless struggle, a Greek myth about Sisyphus pushing a boulder up a hill only to watch it roll back down and then repeat the process for eternity. Because, unlike Sisyphus, Laura found that each time her boulder rolled back down, she learned something new about the hill and herself.

One day, after a while of working together, Laura realised it wasn't about reaching the summit quickly *but about changing her path up the hill*. She started making small, sustainable changes. Instead of crash diets, she found balance in her meals. Instead of infinite cardio sessions, she began walking daily and strength training a few times weekly.

Months and years passed, and Laura's changes stuck. They weren't dramatic, but they were real. One day, she found herself at a summit she had never reached—not because she pushed harder, but because she found a path that worked for her.

This sets the tone nicely for the obstacles and challenges you may have faced throughout your path—starting with a few common ones, such as busy schedules, eating out frequently, and travelling.

Time Management for Busy Schedules

Managing a hectic schedule requires redefining what being fit and healthy means to you. Fitness isn't solely about long gym sessions or strict diets; it's about integrating healthy habits into your daily life. Consider simple adjustments like prioritising quality sleep, reducing alcohol consumption, soaking up some sunlight, taking regular walks, and focusing on your intake of fruits and vegetables. These small choices can significantly improve your overall health over time.

Additionally, if long workouts are daunting, try committing to 15-20 minutes of strength training most days. Alternatively, set a daily step goal that easily integrates into your routine with minimal extra effort. Efficiency is key, not the duration. Use your calendar not just for work and social events but also for scheduling fitness activities. This approach ensures you utilise available moments effectively, leading us nicely on to why planning is crucial.

Planning Ahead

When I was 22, freshly graduated and chilling at my grandmother's place near Croydon, I hit a common post-graduate phase: 3 months of unemployment while job hunting.

A 9-5 job usually brings a routine that can help maintain fitness consistency, thanks to a set daily schedule. So, it was during this period of uncertainty, without a fixed daily routine, that I discovered the real value of planning ahead, and it's a lesson that has stayed with me since.

Effective time management isn't just about finding time; it's about strategically planning to use it wisely. Without a plan, it's easy to fall into the trap of spontaneity, which often leads to inconsistency. Imagine starting your week with the intention to exercise, only to find by Sunday you haven't worked out at all. This scenario is common and highlights the need for a planned approach. Each week, decide in advance which days and times you will dedicate to your workouts—say, Tuesday at 10a.m., Wednesday at 6p.m., and Saturday at 2p.m. By scheduling these sessions as you would any important appointment, you make it far more likely that you'll stick to them.

This planned approach extends beyond exercise to all aspects of a healthy lifestyle, such as meal preparation and ensuring sufficient sleep. By planning these elements, you reinforce your commitment to maintaining fitness, setting the stage for discussing how eating out or grabbing takeaway can fit into this structured approach.

Eating Out or Grabbing Takeaway

Transitioning from the discipline of scheduling workouts and meal planning, let's discuss how to maintain your fitness goals in less controlled scenarios, like dining out.

You've heard the classic statement, "Food is *just* fuel," but I'm afraid I have to disagree. This isn't to say that you shouldn't prioritise healthy, nutritious foods—because, of course, you should. However, this statement completely ignores the fact that food is also a part of culture, religion, celebration, travel and more. It's also a great way to spend time with family and friends.

Food is fuel, but it's also much more than that.

This allows us to appreciate that eating out at restaurants, your aunt's house, or coffee shops is a fun part of life that can bring joy and fulfilment. Enjoying meals out occasionally is perfectly fine; if anything, I'd encourage it. However, if dining out or ordering takeaways is something you do most days, it's essential to be aware that this will likely slow your fat loss progress or perhaps even inhibit it, as you don't have complete control over ingredients like butter, oils, and sauces used in cooking—which is why I'll also often say that cooking at home is an underrated fat loss tip.

Anyway, if you're going out for a meal with friends and you want to plan ahead, or if eating out is something you often do, perhaps due to work, social travel or commitments, or any of the reasons I've named above, and you want to maintain a healthier approach, here are some strategies to consider:

- **Plan Ahead:** If you're visiting a chain restaurant, review their menu in advance and choose options that align with your fitness goals. Many include calorie information.
- **Re-think Dessert:** Instead of always opting for something sweet after, consider a healthier alternative, like fruit salads.
- **Prioritise Lean Protein:** Ensure each meal includes a lean protein source, such as chicken breast, prawns, or tuna.
- **Include Vegetables:** Choose dishes that come with vegetables.
- **Watch Liquid Calories:** Avoid calories from drinks like alcohol and sodas. Consider sticking to water or diet drinks to reduce unnecessary calories.
- **Condiments on the Side:** Request that sauces and dressings be served separately to control the amount you have.

- **Lighter Cooking Requests:** Ask the staff to use less or no oil or butter in your dish. For instance, in Portugal, it's common for them to sometimes add what feels like an ocean of butter to their traditional ham and cheese toasties. So, I'll politely ask them to ease up on the butter whenever I place this order.
- **Choose Smaller Portions:** Have smaller portions when available rather than automatically going for the large.
- **Make Better Choices:** When deciding between fast-food or a healthier location, choose the more nutritious one. If you're at a restaurant, pick the more nutritious meal.
- **Front-Load Protein:** Have at least 30g of protein before going out to eat, and you'll find that you're a lot less hungry. This could come in the form of one or two scoops of protein powder.

This isn't to say that you must implement all of these, as that could be overwhelming. However, consider starting with a few that are manageable for you, especially if frequent meals out are part of your routine.

It could also be worth implementing something I briefly mentioned earlier—bright lines.

Bright lines aren't a specific nutrition approach per se. Instead, think of it as a hard line you draw in a less controlled nutrition environment. When going out to eat, a lot of overeating can typically happen because of a lack of clarity and knowing when and where to stop. However, if you determine your boundaries beforehand, you'll be much more likely to respect them—these are bright lines.

For example, remember when I said it's non-negotiable to have fruit first whenever I want dessert? That's a bright line. Other bright lines for you to consider are forbidding yourself from having more than 2 alcoholic beverages, more than one plate of food for a meal, or stopping eating and drinking after a specific time.

Now, let's move on to a common question I receive: how to maintain your fitness while travelling.

Fitness While Travelling

During a memorable 10-week visit to my girlfriend in Texas, I experienced firsthand the challenges of maintaining fitness while travelling. Transitioning from the walkable cities of Europe to the car-dependent environment of Texas was a significant change. Walking was less practical, and the local cuisine—delicious Texan, Mexican, Japanese, and Vietnamese dishes served in generous portions—was irresistible. Despite keeping up with treadmill walks and gym sessions, the reduced daily activity and colossal portion sizes led to more weight gain than I initially expected.

This journey highlighted the importance of adapting fitness routines to different environments, especially when they massively contrast what you're used to. This experience is a prime example of how a location can influence your fitness goals, a lesson I've learned and now share with you.

When it comes to managing fitness, nutrition, and fat loss during travel, the frequency of your trips plays a crucial role. For those who travel infrequently and mostly for leisure, I suggest a relaxed approach: enjoy your holiday without stressing over fitness or calorie intake. For instance, while I explored cities like Varadero, Montreal, or Nagano, the occasional indulgence was part of the experience. Might you gain a bit of body fat during this period? Potentially, but who cares—the whole reason we're having this coffee shop chat is because you'll know how to lose it once you're back home.

However, if you travel often, whether for pleasure or work, maintaining progress can be challenging due to less control over meals and inconsistent workout routines. Yet, it's still possible to make positive health choices. Utilise hotel gyms, or, like I did while travelling across Europe, secure guest passes at local gyms. Alternatively, a combination of resistance bands and bodyweight exercises can provide a practical workout solution, especially for 15- to 20-minute sessions.

If cooking isn't an option and you must rely on dining out or hotel meals, remember to apply the tips from the previous 'Eating Out or Grabbing Takeaway' section to make healthier choices.

Now that we've covered fitness and nutrition during travel, let's discuss another significant aspect of life that can impact your fitness journey: holiday and festive periods.

Navigating Holidays and Festivities

Transitioning from maintaining fitness while travelling to managing it through the festive season, the challenges continue with a different flavour. The holiday period often brings a unique stress, especially when you're committed to your fat loss goals. Many fear that indulging in holiday festivities might undo months of progress. However, the key lies in your perspective and approach.

Take Christmas as an example. As a Brit with Portuguese roots, I have enjoyed this tradition yearly, except for one year alone in Tokyo. That Christmas, instead of traditional celebrations, I enjoyed local fried chicken and binge-watched "Attack on Titan."

December is notorious for its temptations but managing them is possible with the right mindset. First, understand that your progress isn't dictated by what you do between early December and New Year's; it's dictated by what you do between New Year's and early December.

Second, it's essential to allow some flexibility in your goals. During the holidays, consider shifting your focus from fat loss to either maintenance, accepting you might gain some body fat and aiming to minimise it, or even to performance-based goals in the gym, like achieving a personal best in the barbell squat. This shift helps prevent the holiday season from becoming a source of frustration and allows you to enjoy the celebrations without guilt.

So, here's what you could consider for December:

- **Be Consistent When Not Celebrating:** Christmas Eve, Christmas Day, Boxing Day, a weekly Christmas party and New Year's Eve is *only 8 days, so it isn't an excuse to scrap off an entire month.* You can still do a massive ton on the 23 other days—that's 74% consistency, which is still extremely high considering the time of year.

This consistency could come in the form of:

- **Prioritising Protein:** Ensure your meals have a good protein source.
- **Eating Fruits and Vegetables:** Keep up with your intake of fruits and veggies.
- **Continuing to Walk and Strength Train:** Focus on these not for fat loss but for overall well-being.

Two more messages that are important to leave you with throughout the holiday season are the following:

- **Embrace Imperfection:** Don't set unrealistic goals like never overeating during the holidays. Instead, strive for 'imperfect' actions towards your goals. Be mindful, maintain positive exercise habits, and be kind to yourself if you stray from your plan.
- **Enjoy the Season:** Ultimately, gaining or losing a few pounds over the holidays isn't the end of the world. What matters is that you enjoyed the time. Remember, there's more to life than just your fitness goals. The holiday season is about making memories and enjoying moments with loved ones.

So, as you navigate the festive period, don't view it as a test of perfection. Allow yourself to enjoy the celebrations, be mindful, and remember that a few days won't undo months of progress and consistency.

After discussing the highs of the holiday seasons, let's discuss a crucial topic in health and fitness that often doesn't get the attention it deserves—habits.

Ingrained Habits

When discussing habits, I'd like to share a couple of thoughts. One of the biggest challenges is breaking an ingrained habit, and often, the environment we create for ourselves plays a significant role in our success.

To illustrate this point, let me share a personal story.

Back in 2010, I was 15 years old and addicted to my XBOX360. Like many teenagers in South London, video games were my go-to hobby. Growing up, I spent years on the PlayStation 2 and GameBoy. But by the time I hit secondary school, I switched to the XBOX360. It was a big deal then—most of my friends were playing FIFA, Tekken, and shooting games, and I was hooked.

But here's the problem—I was *really* hooked.

XBOX wasn't just a pastime—it became my life.

After school? XBOX. Weekends? XBOX. Christmas and Easter holidays? XBOX. Friends over? We played XBOX.

Every spare moment was spent hunched in front of that console. While my posture suffered, so did something more valuable: my time. To make matters worse, I wasn't just gaming; I was constantly snacking on junk food—doughnuts, sugary drinks, and chocolate spread sandwiches, all generously supplied by my grandma (you know how grandparents are). My health and well-being were taking a major hit, yet I kept playing.

Gaming with friends wasn't necessarily bad, but looking back, I knew I could have spent my time more wisely—whether focusing on self-improvement, learning something new, or just getting outside more. Even as a teenager, I was aware that I could use my time more effectively.

My dad once told me something that stuck: "You dedicate so much time to it, but when you turn off the console, you're back in the real world with nothing to show for it." At the time, I didn't respond, but that hit hard.

Then one day, something clicked.

After yet another mindless session of career mode on FIFA, accompanied by a pack of doughnuts, I decided enough was enough. I turned off the console, unplugged it, and packed everything into a bag. I put it on a high shelf in my room, out of easy reach.

Here's the interesting part—I didn't ban myself from playing. If I wanted to, I could still get the console, set it up, and play. But now, it required extra effort—more than just pressing a button. That minor inconvenience made all the difference. My gaming habit faded, and I went from hours of daily gaming to not touching it for five years until I eventually gave the console away.

Looking back, I realised my strategy aligned perfectly with James Clear's concept of "Make it Invisible" from *Atomic Habits.* The idea he explains is simple: if you reduce or remove exposure to the cue that triggers a bad habit, the habit itself fades away. The XBOX was my cue, and by making it less accessible, I broke the cycle—not by banning it, but by adding just enough friction to make it less tempting.

Let's say you're trying to eat healthier, but every time you open the cupboard, you see that pack of biscuits staring you in the face. What happens? You give in. But if you remove the temptation—don't buy the biscuits, or store them out of sight—you eliminate the cue, and the habit starts to fade.

On the flip side, James Clear also discusses "Make it Obvious"—a principle for building good habits. To stay consistent, make the cues for your desired habits as visible and accessible as possible. Want to work out more often? Keep your gym clothes in plain sight, or leave your dumbbells next to the TV. When the cue is obvious, the habit becomes easier to maintain.

If you struggle to build good habits in your fitness journey or find it hard to break bad ones, your environment might be holding you back. Perhaps you're trying to lose weight, but your kitchen is stocked with junk food, and your gym clothes are buried at the bottom of your closet. If you want real change, shape your environment to support the habits you want to form.

Another powerful method for building new habits is "habit stacking." James Clear says, "The quickest way to build a new habit into your life is to stack it on top of a current habit." This works because your brain already has a well-established pathway for the existing habit, so adding a new one becomes more effortless.

- After drinking my morning coffee, I'll do a 15-minute workout.
- After brushing my teeth, I'll write 300 words.
- After lunch, I'll take a 10-minute walk.
- After getting into bed, I'll meditate for 3 minutes.
- After showering, I'll apply moisturiser.

Even my teenage habit of eating fried chicken after school in Streatham was an example of habit stacking, though not a healthy one. I had stacked the habit of eating junk food onto the action of finishing my school day. Fortunately, it was a short-lived habit, but it demonstrates how habit stacking can work for both positive and negative outcomes.

Before we move on, I want to leave you with one final thought: small, seemingly insignificant changes may not show any immediate impact, but when you commit to them over time, they can lead to remarkable results.

Now, let's shift our discussion to a different topic: sugar.

Sugar Vilification

Sugar will often get blamed for all the world's problems and more, with many pointing the finger at it for many health issues. But is this vilification of sugar truly necessary?

There's often the debate of whether sugar can genuinely be an addiction, although rather than getting bogged down in semantics, let's speak about the sugar from fruit and then how you can manage your overall sugar intake.

Rethinking Fruit

For some reason, there's this whole issue with fruit.

Freaking fruit.

Some people avoid fruit due to its sugar content, fearing fat gain. Of course, too much of anything could potentially result in excess calories, which would lead to fat gain. However, realise this: How many people have gotten fat from eating too many strawberries, melons, kiwis, mangos, or oranges? It just doesn't happen. Fruit isn't even close to being in the top 200 issues for fitness and obesity, and people who claim it should be avoided because of its sugar content are doing infinitely more harm than good. Fruit is loaded with nutrients and fibre, making it a beneficial part of any diet.

If anyone tells you that you should stop eating fruit because the sugar in it will make you fat, never take nutrition advice from that person again.

Managing Sugar Intake

Excessive sugar intake from more "fun foods" can potentially lead to health problems, but moderation is key. Here are some strategies to manage sugar consumption effectively:

- Avoid stocking up on sugary treats to reduce temptation. If you can't do this due to family or housemates, make these items less accessible, like storing them on the highest shelf (like I did with my XBOX).
- Go for single-serving sizes of treats instead of family-sized packs. This adds a barrier to overeating because if you want more, that's fine; however, you'll have to take a trip to the store.
- Incorporate tactics discussed earlier, like the 20-minute wait rule or choosing fruits, salads or protein-rich snacks first.

- Ultimately, remember that you are in control of your food choices. Saying no and making choices aligned with your goals might be challenging initially. Still, it becomes easier with time and repetition.

In summary, while sugar is often vilified—ironically over foods that almost always combine sugar with fats and salts to create an irresistible taste, not sugar in isolation—it's important to understand its role in a balanced diet. In the same way one hot day doesn't make a summer (unless you live in the north of England), ice cream once in a while can be enjoyed as part of a well-balanced diet. Remember, moderation, not elimination, is the approach that brings enjoyment to life and health.

This nicely brings up 2 of the most overrated terms within the fitness space: cheat meals and cheat days.

Cheat Meals and Cheat Days

If your fitness plan includes "cheat meals" or "cheat days", then chances are, it's not a very good one.

Let me explain.

Firstly, think about what "cheating" implies. What are you "cheating" on? Your diet? If so, it's worth rethinking your nutrition plan. A good nutritional approach shouldn't make you feel restricted to the point of needing to "cheat".

Second, the origin of these terms lies in the bodybuilding world, where extreme discipline in diet and training is essential for competition day. On this day, competitors strive to be at an unhealthy and unsustainable level of body fat percentage so that they can strip down and pose to the judges to flaunt the physique they've worked on.

However, for you, who is aiming for general fat loss and muscle gain, this approach is entirely unnecessary. Implementing "cheat days" or "cheat meals" can only be a red flag.

Now, this isn't to say that you shouldn't be consistent with what you eat and drink because, of course, that's vital in achieving your fat loss goals. One strategy I often recommend to my 1-2-1 online fitness members who track calories is encouraging "untracked meals" wherever it makes sense. This can accommodate social events like birthdays or weddings, helping to maintain long-term diet sustainability. Plus, the wording from a psychological perspective can and will make all the difference.

However, dedicating a whole meal or day to binge eating, which is essentially what cheat meals and days are, and then returning to a rigorous diet is just a binge-restrict cycle with a fancy name.

A final point to consider is the restriction of certain foods.

Often, cheat meals happen because of the banning of specific food groups. If you don't impose such bans, you won't feel the urge to "cheat". I suggest somewhat following the 80/20 guideline: get 80% of your calories from nutritious, single-ingredient foods, and allow 20% for the rest, like the tempting sugar-coated doughnut you've been eyeing.

Persisting with Previous Methods

Perhaps one of the most common fat loss journey mistakes, which can potentially make daily life more challenging, is the persistence to stick with a fitness routine that served you well at one point in life but no longer works for where you are now.

Understand that what worked well for you 5 years ago, or even 6 months ago, might not be ideal today. Perhaps earlier, you had more free time, fewer responsibilities, or different daily habits. Now, your situation might have evolved; you could have a full-time job, a child, different financial circumstances, or less time for physical activity.

This reluctance to change regarding fitness and fat loss could be tied to the sunk-cost fallacy, a concept my mate Akim introduced when we were teenagers. He explained the sunk-cost fallacy to me as to why people sometimes continue in relationships even though they're no longer working out, simply because they've already invested a lot of time, effort, and money into them. It's a common trap that can hinder progress in various aspects of life, including your health and fitness journey. Recognising the sunk-cost fallacy at play can empower you to make necessary changes, even if it means abandoning a method in which you've heavily invested.

Remember that your body and environment are constantly changing. You must learn how to adapt to them. Sticking to outdated routines can lead to frustration and stagnation. You might need to figure out new methods and apply them, such as implementing what you've learned and will continue to learn from throughout this chat.

Now, to continue with the theme of common weight loss challenges, let's discuss perhaps the biggest of all—fat loss plateaus.

Chapter 11:
Fat Loss Plateaus

First, it's crucial to understand that not seeing a change in your scale weight, measurements or progress pictures after a week isn't a plateau. True plateaus require up to about 3 weeks of consistent effort without change to confirm a plateau, not 3 days. So, if you've barely been consistent, it's only been a couple of weeks, or both; I can confirm that you're not in a plateau, just yet.

Having said that, eventually hitting a plateau is also a standard part of any journey, whether in fat loss, learning a new language, or improving at chess. When you've been working hard at something for a while, you likely reach a point where progress stalls. It's normal and often a sign that you've made significant progress already. So, if you've hit a plateau in your fat loss journey, give yourself a pat on the back for the hard work you've put in so far!

Now, let's discuss why fat loss plateaus occur. There are many potential reasons, but I'll focus on a few common ones and what you can do about them.

Inaccuracies

When I say inaccuracies, I specifically mean those related to tracking food and scale weight, as these are common mistakes I've often encountered in my career. Both factors are critical in managing your fitness journey and getting them right can significantly impact your progress or how you perceive things to be going.

Calorie Tracking

Calorie tracking can be a fantastic tool for many people. Still, its effectiveness depends on how accurately you log your food. A common mistake for beginners is relying on eyeballing and guesstimation to determine portion sizes.

This approach, to be straight-up, is unreliable. Suppose you're new to tracking your food and drink intake. How can you accurately estimate what 100 grams of rice, a tablespoon of peanut butter, or the exact weight of a beef serving is? You cannot. Seemingly minor errors in estimation can add up massively over time, leading to big miscalculations in your weekly calorie count.

I saw this firsthand with Hakeem, a 1-2-1 online fitness member from South London, estate agent, and an Arsenal FC fan. He initially relied on guesswork for his food tracking. After noticing inconsistencies in his data, I suggested he use a kitchen scale and measuring jug for 30 days to improve his accuracy.

Here's his first message the next day: "I can't believe that's what 100g of rice looks like!"

Though Hakeem wasn't keen on continuing with calorie tracking after the 30 days, that month of precise measurement was an eye-opener and set him up for lasting success. Suppose you find yourself in a similar situation. In that case, I recommend a period of diligent, accurate tracking to truly understand the size and caloric content of your meals—chances are, it'll likely reveal some surprises.

Bites, Licks and Nibbles

An often-overlooked aspect is bites, licks, and nibbles. These seemingly insignificant eating habits that you don't think twice about might seem harmless in the moment, but they can quietly contribute to stalling fat loss progress.

So, what are these 'bites, licks, and nibbles'? Here are a few everyday examples:

- Half a glass of the new orange juice at breakfast adds around 55 calories.
- Accepting a chocolate finger offered by a colleague at work, which is about 50 calories.
- Having a few bites of a doughnut while watching television adds up to around 90 calories.
- Unconsciously grabbing a handful of nuts during our coffee shop chat can be upwards of 200 calories.
- Finishing off half of your child's ice cream after school, about 110 calories.
- Spreading butter on your toast, where the quantity is often underestimated, leads to around 200 calories.
- Sampling a few spoonfuls of your partner's rice at dinner is approximately 50 calories.

Of course, occasionally experiencing this won't derail your progress, but consistently overlooking these calories will add up, especially over weeks or months. This gradual accumulation can be the reason behind a frustrating plateau in your fat loss journey, so it's worth being attentive.

Scale Weight

Regarding scale weight, the key to accuracy is consistency in how and when you take your readings. I'll properly touch on this topic later. Still, it's worth briefly mentioning the importance of consistent conditions for weigh-ins. Your weight can fluctuate considerably throughout the day due to various factors like food intake, hydration levels, and even bowel movements.

For the most consistent results, weigh yourself in a fasted state first thing in the morning after using the bathroom. This provides a baseline that is as consistent as possible. For example, I remember a day when my weight dropped by 0.4kg just from a morning bathroom visit, only to increase by nearly a kilogram after drinking 500ml of water—all within 5 minutes.

Here's how it went:

- 7:38a.m. (wake up) – 81.2 kg
- 7:41a.m. (post-urination) – 80.8 kg
- 7:43a.m. (post-500ml of water) – 81.7 kg

These fluctuations illustrate why weighing yourself randomly throughout the day can lead to misleading readings.

Your Body Has Adapted

This brings us to the common myth of "starvation mode." Many believe that eating too little can lead to weight gain, but that's simply not true—it's like suggesting a plant will grow more by depriving it of water and sunlight.

Let's use the Minnesota starvation experiment as an example.

This study was conducted at the University of Minnesota from November 19, 1944, until December 20, 1945. Although ethically questionable by today's standards, this study aimed to understand the effects of severe, prolonged dietary restriction. The result? Participants significantly lost weight, debunking the idea that eating too little leads to weight gain. If starvation mode were real, these people would have gained body fat, which wasn't the case. They inevitably ended up extremely underweight due to the lack of food.

So what really happens when people say "your body has adapted" is actually something called metabolic adaptation, *which is different*:

- As you reduce your calorie intake, your body may respond by conserving energy. You might move less without realising it, such as fidgeting, pacing less, or even being less animated when speaking.
- As you lose weight, your body naturally becomes more efficient at using calories. Thus, you require fewer calories to do the same activities.
- If you lose muscle mass along with fat—particularly if you're not doing strength training or eating enough protein—your metabolism might slow down. Remember when I said that muscle tissue burns more calories at rest than fat tissue?

Now, to clarify the difference between starvation mode and metabolic adaptation:

- **Starvation mode** (false) claims that eating too little causes weight *gain*.
- **Metabolic adaptation** (true) means your body *requires fewer calories* after a period of dieting, slowing weight loss—but it never causes you to gain weight just from eating less.

Remember, your body aims for homeostasis, which means maintaining a stable internal environment, including weight. These adaptations are simply your body's way of trying to keep you in balance—and they're perfectly normal. Understanding this can help you stay on track as you move forward in your fat loss journey, without feeling frustrated by the natural changes your body undergoes.

Becoming More Intentional

First, it's essential to clarify the term newbie gains. This is the rapid progress in your fitness, strength and muscle growth that people often experience when working out for the first time—even with a poorly structured workout plan. I'll sometimes jokingly say that throughout this phase, you can simply look at a barbell and make progress.

When your body isn't used to lifting weights or exercising, it responds quickly and dramatically, making gains faster at the beginning of your fitness journey than it will later once your body has become more accustomed to the workouts. Once this initial phase is over, you'll need to ensure you're more intentional with your approach to continue making progress.

Although the brief story I'm about to share isn't specifically fat loss related and instead has more to do with workouts, an illustration of this concept occurred while I was working at a gym in Fulham.

There was a gym member, let's call her Debby, who was puzzled about not seeing the same progress she once did despite regularly attending gym classes. Initially, Debby saw significant improvements from consistently attending gym classes because she went from zero to regular exercise—this was her experiencing the 'newbie gains' phase.

However, after this initial phase of newbie gains, she needed a more personalised training approach to ensure progressive overload if she wanted to continue progressing. While gym classes can be a decent starting place, they don't consider the individual, which is necessary for continued progress—mainly because they don't build on each other in a structured way.

So, like Debby, as you've become fitter and healthier, your journey now demands a higher level of planning or consistency to reach the next level. What worked for you initially when starting from scratch might be less effective now that you've progressed to a fitter and healthier version of yourself. Perhaps you must be more intentional with specific factors in your approach, too, such as tracking your workouts, calories or steps.

Psychological Factors

Psychological factors like fading motivation or lower adherence to your diet and exercise plan should also be considered. We've touched on motivation already, so revisiting those sections for a refresher might be helpful. However, a gradual decline in consistency is more common than you might think. In fact, many people often overestimate how consistent they are; this could be true for you, too. Initially, you might have been incredibly consistent, but as you began to see results, you might have become more lenient.

Picture this: Imagine you've tied a big ship to the shore. Every day, several times a day, you check to make sure it's still tightly secured. But as time goes by, you start to check less often and from further away, not noticing the ropes are gradually loosening. Eventually, you stop checking, and one day, you take a peep and see the ship is gone.

This analogy, shared with me in a conversation with psychologist Dr. Josh Smith, mirrors how people's commitment can gradually erode over time.

It reminds me of Maeve, an Irish gym-goer at that same Fulham gym where I worked, who shared her struggles with me. She mentioned that whenever she progressed in her fitness and fat loss, she'd become more lenient and "treat herself to her favourite dark chocolate a lot more than usual". Based on my experience, it's likely that not just the chocolate but perhaps a decrease in activities like walking and enjoying other snacks more frequently also contributed to this pattern.

This relaxation in her routine was like the ship's ropes loosening, leading to a cycle she describes as "the same progression and regression."

Regardless of where you feel you're at with this one, I'd suggest using a consistency calendar tool that we'll touch on later to measure what you're doing. It could also be worth considering if you're perhaps initially being overly rigid when starting your fitness routine, to the point you feel the need to overeat foods you previously wouldn't allow, contributing to this frustrating cycle.

You're Not in a Plateau

Let me take you back to one autumn.

I was having a call with Laura, the same 1-2-1 online fitness member I mentioned earlier. She shared her frustrations, saying, "Leo, I love my training, but I feel like I've hit a plateau in my fat loss, and it's getting demotivating."

I was surprised—not by her openness, which I always love, but by her statement, because she wasn't actually plateauing at all.

"Why do you feel like that?" I asked. "Your data shows an average weekly weight loss of 0.5kg, and your measurements have consistently been on a downward trend."

She realised and chuckled, "Oh yeah, you're right. I guess I was just in my head about it. Sorry!"

Our conversation continued, covering her future fitness plans, lovely cat, and the scarce sunlight in Oslo during winter.

Her confusion made sense, though. After a five-week intense fat loss phase we'd done earlier in the year, her current steady progress seemed slow in comparison. Comparing an unusually rapid phase with normal, steady improvement is an easy mistake.

I share this story because with all of this said, you might not even be in a plateau.

As I mentioned, when you start a fitness regime, your body rapidly responds to new challenges, like quickly advancing through the initial levels of a new video game. This phase is exciting; you learn new skills, build confidence, and see noticeable progress. However, as you advance, like the game's later levels, improvement becomes more challenging and demands greater skill and strategy.

Perhaps your initial methods for strength training, fitness, or fat loss led to quick results, but as you lean down, progress naturally slows down because you have less body fat to lose.

The key here is to understand that your rate of progress is perhaps still on track for both muscle gain and fat loss. However, your perception of reasonable progress may have been slightly skewed by unrealistic expectations from the marketing world, social media, the rapid advancements during the newbie gains phase, or like Laura, more aggressive approaches you've previously used. Adjusting your expectations to align with your current stage in your fat loss journey is vital. What you might perceive as a plateau could be the progression of your body naturally responding more slowly to current efforts.

So, remember, it's not unusual for progress to appear to slow down. This doesn't mean you've hit a wall; it's just an indication that your journey is evolving and that you're in a new chapter. Continue to be dedicated. In the worst-case scenario, perhaps an adjustment or two will be eventually required—either way, you'll be fine.

Overcoming Plateaus

As you'll know by now, overcoming plateaus is a normal part of a fat loss journey. You might wonder what the next step is—whether it's increasing your steps, ramping up cardio, cutting calories, or boosting your protein intake.

First, ensure your consistency is solid; if you've barely been consistent, you have no right to complain about a lack of results or being in a plateau—you need to work on that first.

Second, it's worth realising that if you're never hungry and have been in a plateau for several weeks, you're likely not in a calorie deficit. Feeling constantly starved or obsessively thinking about food all day indicates an unnecessarily aggressive deficit, which I wouldn't recommend. However, being in a reasonable deficit will likely sometimes involve some slight hunger occasionally, usually before meals or bedtime.

Third, it's vital to have previously tracked, too, such as workouts, nutrition, steps, sleep, etc. You know what they say: *what gets measured gets managed*. This data helps identify what potentially needs adjusting.

Any good scientist will tell you that changing only one variable at a time is crucial when conducting a study or experiment. If you change too many variables at once, you won't know what was previously at fault, slowing you down or which change worked for you. This can also be a similar situation during a plateau.

While I can't offer tailored advice without more specific context, the general approach, as mentioned, is to make 1 or 2 changes, like tweaking caloric intake, improving sleep quality, increasing daily steps, starting strength training, eating more fibre and protein, etc. Then, stay consistent with this adjustment for a few weeks to gauge its effectiveness. Throwing the kitchen sink during a plateau will only cause further challenges and likely slow you down more.

That said, let's discuss one of the most overlooked factors in a fitness journey: your environment.

Chapter 12:
The Role of Community and Environment

An often-overlooked aspect of your fitness journey, and even life in general, is the influence of the people and environments around you. Of course, this includes people you'll go to coffee shops with, such as myself. Still, it also includes family, friends, work colleagues, coaches, teachers, mentors, and broader communities, right up to societal norms that vary from country to country, each with unique expectations and challenges.

The power of community is enormous and will significantly impact you positively or negatively, with effects that go well beyond fitness.

After all, you know the saying from Jim Rohn: *"You are the average of the 5 people you spend the most time with."*

Consider these examples:

- Schoolmates with top grades falling into hard drugs simply by associating with the wrong crowd.
- Polyglots consistently joining group calls to communicate with others who speak the language they're learning, hugely boosting their skills.
- My 1-2-1 online fitness members benefiting from the support and motivation of other like-minded members on their fitness journey.

- Members of my local BJJ dojo consistently push each other towards improvement—slowly increasing their skill as time passes.
- Friends who were once fitness enthusiasts completely altering their lifestyle, neglecting their health after partnering with someone uninterested in working out.
- My business mentors bring together a community to bounce inspiration and motivation amongst their members.
- Drinkers struggling to quit because it's all their social circle does.

Realising how these communities and environments impact you is crucial.

It's clear that some of these social scenarios are easier to influence and adjust than others, so this part of our chat isn't to dictate what you should or shouldn't do. Instead, it's about raising awareness of the dynamics in your social environment and how they might affect your fitness journey and overall well-being.

For example, suppose you're continuously around people with a fixed mindset (remember what we discussed in the psychology section?). In that case, you'll have a much more challenging time making progress and a lower likelihood of reaching your goal.

Let's expand on several key areas, including partners, peer pressure, community, and more.

Partners and Close Friends

As mentioned, your partner and close friends can play a big role in your fitness and fat loss journey—positive or negative. They might say they're supportive, but sometimes, perhaps subconsciously, they might act in ways that sabotage your fitness goals. This might happen because they see you changing—like getting stronger at the gym or losing inches around your waist—and feel bad about themselves for not making similar changes. So, instead of making positive changes, they opt for the easier option to try and keep things the way they were—which is to hold you back.

It's important to consider whether this person really supports your health and fitness goals. Compare how they treated you at the start of your relationship to how they treat you now. Would you still have dated or befriended them if they acted this way initially?

People often stay in jobs they don't like or relationships and friendships they're not interested in because they fear change. When they're not happy with many other parts of their daily lives, they might then turn to food because it's the one thing that brings excitement to their day. I know it's messed up, but it's true.

I'm not saying you should end things with these people either—I understand it's not always that simple. But it's essential to be aware of these dynamics. They're more common than you might think, and you might be experiencing them, too.

Now that we've looked at how your partner can impact your fitness and fat loss goals, let's talk about how to deal with pressure from other people around you.

Peer Pressure

Remember Alex, my online fitness member and avid Benfica fan who lives in Portugal? The location means he enjoys great weather and cuisine most of the year, but this also means frequent social events and the accompanying pressure to often overindulge in food and drink.

I've always emphasised the importance of enjoying life's pleasures, including social gatherings. However, excessive indulgence can stall your progress, especially if done regularly. Alex understood this balance well.

When he started his healthy lifestyle, Alex faced significant peer pressure from friends who always urged him to eat or drink more, making it challenging to stay committed. I advised him that while it might feel difficult, it's essential to remember that not everyone will understand his health goals, and it's okay to politely decline.

Following that, I then suggested several strategies for managing these situations:

- **Just Say 'No':** It may be challenging initially, but saying 'No, thank you' gets easier with practice. It sounds obvious, but sometimes it doesn't need to be overcomplicated. You're in control of your diet, and there's no need to justify your choices.

- **The 'Challenge' Excuse:** Claiming you're in the middle of a personal challenge, like avoiding alcohol for 50 days or skipping dessert for a month, often makes people back off. The specifics don't matter as much as the principle of setting boundaries—it doesn't have to be true either. The main aim is to get the person to stop bugging you. You might be surprised at how well this one works.

- **Accept and Delay:** If someone insists on you having a treat, accept it but plan to enjoy it later—for example, if you're at a restaurant, then take it to go. Remember, you don't have to eat everything immediately.

- **Avoid Discussing Your Diet:** When pressured to share food or eat more, a simple 'I'm good, thanks' is enough. Refrain from engaging in lengthy justifications or debates about your food choices.

- **Stay in Control:** Ultimately, you decide what you eat and drink. Yes, occasional slip-ups happen because you're human. However, it's your responsibility to stay consistent with your health goals.

Alex adopted some of these strategies, improving his ability to balance health, exercise, social events, beer and great food!

This success is also partly due to another crucial factor—holding himself accountable. Many people struggle with their health and fitness because they perceive external factors as controlling their outcomes. Alex made progress by recognising that he had control over his responses to these situations.

Think: Even though external reasons for your struggle may be valid, what now?

Not every day will be a good day for fat loss and fitness, but blaming others or circumstances outside your control isn't a helpful way to think.

For example, when I lose a chess game, get submitted in BJJ, or get knocked out of a poker game, I think about what I can do differently next time. I ask myself how I can improve or change my approach.

There's always at least one thing in your control that you can tackle. *Focus on that.*

Plus, and I'm sure you can relate when I say that pursuing fat loss and fitness goals is a journey that others might not always understand or support. It's crucial to recognise that any negativity you encounter from others likely reflects their potential issues, not a problem with what you're working towards.

If you know that improving your health, shedding body fat, and gaining strength will transform you into a better version of yourself, for your children, friends, family, and partners, then fight for it, and don't feel bad. Alex knew.

Next up: community.

Community

Staying consistent with exercise is easier when you're not doing it alone. Now, I'll expand on coaches, mentors, and teachers shortly. However, having other people around you, like friends, who are also serious about their fitness goals and are on a similar mission, can make a big difference. This is a big reason why groups like CrossFit are so successful—they use the power of community. People enjoy being around others who share their ambitions.

My personal story highlights how valuable this community aspect can be.

One spring, while at Bishop Thomas Grant Sixth Form (BTG) in London, I was part of a BTEC in Sport course. During one phase of this two-year course, we had a particular module focused on strength training and cardio, which was fascinating, especially since I had only started going to the gym about a year or so beforehand.

Our school gave us memberships to the FitnessFirst (FF) in Streatham, and our class would go there twice a week. It was a small class going to FF, 8 to be precise, 4 guys and 4 girls, and under the supervision of Miss Andrews, our workouts weren't just about exercising; they ended up being about supporting each other—especially with the comradery us 4 guys developed the more we went. We all helped one another, shared tips, and even took the piss out of each other in the best way possible.

Training together had a kind of magic to it. We pushed each other to go further than we thought we could, creating a bond and a sense of motivation that's hard to find when you're working out alone. This experience showed me how great a supportive community is for making progress.

Years later, this lesson about the power of community still sticks with me. I aim to incorporate it into my 1-2-1 online fitness coaching, too.

So, if you're feeling stuck right now, perhaps it could be time to find a gym buddy. However, it's also vital that you don't solely rely on them either because you don't want 100% of your workouts to depend on whether or not they'll flake on you. So, ensure you get it done regardless, and think of having them by your side as a lovely bonus.

With partners, peer pressure and community having been discussed. Let's cover microculture.

Microculture

There's a crucial element in your environment called "microculture"—the culture within your household. It's an unseen force that influences what you eat, how you behave, and the choices you make, subtly shaping your actions even when you think you're making decisions freely.

Taking control of your microculture can significantly impact your fitness journey, especially by reducing how often you need to rely on willpower.

I often hear people struggling with fitness goals say, 'I just wish I had more willpower like Amy.' However, Amy's success likely has more to do with how she structures her environment to reduce the need for willpower. It's a common misconception that successful fat loss requires superhuman willpower. In reality, many who have lost body fat and kept it off do so by optimising their surroundings, not just relying on discipline.

Structuring your environment to support your goals makes the journey less about constant self-control and more about setting yourself up for success. To illustrate the power of the environment, let's consider the extreme situation of American soldiers in Vietnam.

Many soldiers, surrounded by the harsh realities of war and with easy access to high-quality, inexpensive heroin, developed addictions. The U.S. government feared a heroin epidemic when these soldiers returned home, expecting a surge in addiction-related issues—costing millions of dollars and flooding hospitals. However, contrary to expectations, only 5% of the returning soldiers relapsed into heroin use, a stark contrast to the typical 90% relapse rate.

The key factor? A change in environment.

When the soldiers returned to the U.S., they were removed from the stress, idle time, and peer influence in Vietnam. The environmental cues associated with drug use were no longer present, which significantly reduced the urge to use heroin. While this is an extreme example, it highlights the profound impact of our surroundings on behaviour, shaping positive and negative habits alike.

When building healthy habits, adjusting your environment can make or break your success. Here are a few practical strategies to create a home environment that supports your fitness goals:

- **Limit Temptations:** Keep less healthy foods out of the house, or if that's not feasible, make them less accessible (e.g., in a cupboard that's hard to reach).

- **Stock Nutritious Foods:** Keep healthy options like fruit visible, such as in a fruit bowl on the kitchen counter.
- **Mindful Eating:** Reduce screen time during meals to promote mindfulness, helping you be more aware of what and how much you're eating.
- **Portion Control:** Serve snacks in a bowl rather than eating straight from the packet to better manage portions. Eating directly from the packet can blur the line of when to stop, while using a bowl provides a clear endpoint—once it's empty, you're done.
- **Reduce Liquid Calories:** Minimise sugary drinks in the house and replace them with water, diet soda, or healthier options.

Optimising your home environment can significantly boost your success, making healthy choices feel natural rather than forced. Now, let's explore how coaches, mentors, and teachers can further support your journey.

Coaches, Mentors and Teachers

When I was 17, I was dropped from sixth form, leaving me lost and uncertain about my future. During this low point, two wonderful teachers I knew personally—Madalena, a Portuguese woman, and Kathleen, a Colombian—noticed my struggle. In their free time, they had a heart-to-heart conversation with me at BTG, the sixth form I eventually joined. That moment became a turning point, setting me back on a productive path and helping me clarify my future.

While 'coach,' 'mentor,' and 'teacher' may sometimes be used interchangeably, each plays a distinct role. Teachers primarily share knowledge and skills in an educational setting, mentors provide guidance and wisdom based on their own experiences, and coaches excel in working towards specific personal or professional goals. While the three roles overlap to an extent, they each play a vital role in learning and development.

The accountability and inspiration coaches, mentors, and teachers provide (I'll refer to all 3 as "guides") can be the difference maker. Having someone to report to and hold you accountable drastically increases your chances of maintaining consistency.

This is especially effective in fitness and fat loss.

If you want to make consistent progress, hiring a coach could be one of the smartest moves you can make.

You might think, 'Well, Leo, you're a fitness coach; of course you'd say that!'

But here's my perspective: I chose to become a coach because I've experienced firsthand the value they add. I've sought accountability whenever I've aspired to improve significantly at something.

- To boost my strength and fitness, I hired an online fitness coach.
- When improving my Japanese, I paid a language teacher for weekly lessons.
- I signed up with a mentor for business growth who set regular tasks and goals.
- Paid for a yearly membership at my local BJJ dojo to reap the benefits of having excellent BJJ coaches.

Thanks to these professionals' accountability, my progress and consistency skyrocketed in each case.

A common response I often hear is, 'Leo, I already know what I need to do, so I don't need someone to keep me accountable. Besides, I can find everything I need online for free.'

Okay, perhaps you know what you must do, but consider this: Knowledge alone, and merely having access to resources online, isn't enough. *It's the application that counts.*

Have you been applying it?

How has that been working for you so far?

Why did you decide to entertain this chat with me for this long if this is the case?

You can know precisely what you need to do, but application is a whole other ball game—and one you might not be on top of.

Accountability can be transformative. It stems from not wanting to disappoint those you've turned to for guidance or wasting your investment in yourself. Not having this external accountability could be what's holding you back. Moreover, guides often provide inspiration, especially during challenging phases in life. Having such influential and experienced figures in your corner isn't just beneficial—it's game-changing.

Now that we've discussed one of the pivotal factors that will help you progress, let's move on to something that will help you recognise whether you're on the right track.

Chapter 13:
Indicators of Progress

Imagine, as we reach the last sips of our coffee, noticing the patterns left by the foam on the inside of the mug—and each one, according to Turkish coffee fortune-telling, tells a unique story. Now, I must admit, I've never looked into Turkish coffee fortune-telling beyond simply hearing about it, but I bring this up because, similarly, your journey in fat loss has unique ways of showing your story and the progress you've made up until now.

Understanding how to track your progress effectively can be the difference between giving up and continuing your fat loss journey. Relying solely on the scale to measure your success is a common mistake. So, with that, let's get stuck into potential indicators.

Scale Weight

While I spoke against relying solely on the scale, it can still be great when used correctly. For the most accurate readings, weigh yourself at the same time each day, preferably upon waking up, after using the bathroom, in a fasted state, and preferably wearing the same clothes, or as I'll do, while just wearing underwear. This helps minimise the impact of external variables on your weight.

Recording your weight regularly and taking weekly averages allows a more accurate view of your progress as it accounts for daily fluctuations. I say this because I've seen scale weight differ by as much as 4 to 5kg within the same week. Consider the following example from my first week in September:

Monday: 82kg
Tuesday: 82.8kg
Wednesday: 81.8kg
Thursday: 82.4kg
Friday: 82.4kg
Saturday: 82.1kg
Sunday: 82.3kg

This means my average weight for week one of September is 82.3 kg, removing any inconsistencies from any unusual fluctuations. Imagine if you didn't weigh yourself daily and take a weekly average. You could have weighed yourself only on Tuesday when your weight was the highest, gotten frustrated, and given up.

Fluctuations can occur due to hormones, hydration levels, food, whether you need to use the toilet, a heavy weightlifting session the day before, and more. So, contrary to popular belief, the scale is not just measuring fat.

It's also important to acknowledge that if you don't feel psychologically ready to weigh yourself frequently, or it makes you feel super anxious, then that's okay too—you don't have to take scale weight. You can look at other indicators, which brings us nicely to measurements.

Body Measurements

Body measurements are excellent and an underrated indicator of progress, particularly for fat loss. Measuring areas—such as the widest part of your hips, around your belly button, and a consistent spot on your thigh—can reveal changes you might not notice by just using the scale. These measurements can sometimes show progress even when your weight remains constant, and vice versa. This is also why I recommend tracking several indicators of progress at once.

I suggest taking measurements bi-weekly, under the same conditions as your weigh-ins: in the morning, in a fasted state, and after using the bathroom. This consistency ensures that the changes you see are due to your approach rather than external factors—like the fact you've just eaten a massive lunch.

Progress Pictures

When my 1-2-1 online fitness member and friend, Anca, started working with me, she was initially hesitant with taking progress pictures—often taking low-effort selfies in which she'd hide her face, hunched over, while wearing baggy clothes. Fast forward one year later, after making tremendous strides with her progress, the difference is enormous. Not only is she noticeably leaner and stronger, but she puts much more effort into taking these pictures, wearing tighter sports clothes, an upright posture and a smile on her now visible face—all a fantastic reminder that progress isn't just physical.

I understand that taking your first set of progress pictures can feel daunting. However, I'm yet to meet someone who's made significant progress and regrets taking their first set of pictures. *I've only met people who regret not getting that first shot.* Even Anca says she regrets not taking her progress pictures sooner. Progress pictures are a powerful tool for seeing changes that are otherwise easy to overlook, especially when it's easy to feel like daily or weekly actions may not have much to show.

Comparing photos from long enough periods, like January to September, can often reveal massive changes, providing a lovely motivational boost.

For a consistent view, capture front, back, and side shots. Even casual gym selfies or snapshots from social events can reveal progress unexpectedly when compared to older photos.

Regarding frequency, aiming for monthly pictures offers a consistent timeline, while, at a minimum, every 3 months can still be a strong amount.

Old Clothes and Watch Straps

In addition to photos, the fit of old clothes and the adjustment of watch straps serve as valid, though less common, indicators of progress.

Perhaps there was a moment when your favourite pair of jeans became uncomfortably tight, and you realised the need for change. Fast forward 6 months of consistent effort toward your fat loss goals, and those same jeans now fit comfortably, just as they did in your favourite memories of them.

Similarly, a watch that once fit at a particular lug hole might now require tightening due to a reduced wrist size—another subtle yet significant sign of progress.

Such changes, though small, are concrete evidence of your transformation and deserve recognition.

Improved Habits

Improved habits are vital for any successful fat loss journey. While it may not seem as exciting as physical transformations, recognising and celebrating the consistency in healthier habits is essential. Remember, progress in a fitness journey isn't limited to what you can see; it also includes behavioural changes that ultimately lead you to your desired outcome.

As mentioned earlier in our chat, improved habits and a stronger mindset lead to lasting results. Anyone can lose weight quickly, but keeping it off forever requires these permanent changes.

Improved habits can come in various forms, such as:

- Reducing nightly beer consumption from 3 every night to one every other day.
- Opting to walk to the local shop instead of driving.
- Incorporating more protein into your breakfast, moving away from a carb and fat-heavy start to the day.
- Overcoming the initial fear of the gym and starting to enjoy your workouts.
- Swapping the family-sized bag of cookies for fruit as your go-to snack.

Noticing an improvement in your habits can be incredibly motivating. Using tools, such as the consistency calendar, which I'll explain to you shortly, to track these small victories can help visualise your consistency and progress, potentially resulting in even more motivation!

For example, when I focused on improving my Japanese language skills, setting a goal of completing 6 related tasks weekly massively boosted my consistency. Whether engaging in a language exchange call, filling out a page in my textbook, or watching a video on the subject, seeing these 6 weekly tasks accumulate over time made me want to keep going.

Similarly, you might set a goal for daily water intake, such as drinking at least one litre daily. Seeing this habit become a part of your routine contributes to your health and reinforces your new identity as someone committed to your well-being.

This talk on habits nicely brings us onto the consistency calendar—a valuable tool for habit-tracking progress.

Consistency Calendar

One cloudy day in Fulham—typical weather for the area—I was working as a personal trainer on the gym floor when Tony approached me. Although we hadn't spoken much before, Tony, a friendly man in his late 30s who worked a full-time office job, had a question he seemed eager to ask.

"Hey, how's it going?" he started, then quickly got into his concern. "I'm struggling to make progress in my fat loss journey, and I can't figure out where I'm going wrong."

After a few questions and some thought, I offered a suggestion that might help. "Tony, have you ever considered using a consistency calendar for just 30 days?" I explained that a consistency calendar is an excellent tool for accurately tracking adherence to daily goals because it's common to overestimate one's consistency.

And based on what he'd said, I suspected Tony might be overestimating his own.

Here's how the consistency calendar works:
For each day you meet your goals—let's say it's sticking to your calorie intake, reaching your step count, and completing workouts where applicable—mark it with a check (✔). On days when you fall short in any one of these areas, mark it with a circle (O). Aim for a consistency range of 85-95% by the end of the month—I find this is the sweet spot between fitness progress and balancing a social life.

If you fall below this range, it's a clear indicator that there's room to improve.

Tony was open to trying the consistency calendar, and interestingly, just over 30 days later, he shared an eye-opening realisation. While working out at the gym, he approached me, saying, "Leo, you were right. I used Friday, Saturday, and Sunday as more of a 'break' than I realised. I thought I was just a few calories over, but it was closer to 1,000 each day. Tracking it on the calendar really made me mindful!"

This scenario isn't uncommon. The "ease up on the weekend" mentality affects many. Weekends, including Friday, make up 43% of your month. That's a lot. And you cannot get 85-95% type fitness results from 57% consistency. The consistency calendar helped highlight this for Tony.

This lesson from the consistency calendar was a turning point, prompting him to focus on winning the weekends to continue progressing.

Before moving on to discussing strength gains, I want to mention two more things.

The first is that your inconsistency might not necessarily be from the weekend; it could happen anytime within the month.

The second is that I mentioned 85-95% consistency is the sweet spot because it's essential to acknowledge that inconsistent days aren't all bad. Having a few days where you relax with your regimen is healthy. This doesn't mean eat everything in sight, but more because it might be due to a social meal out, a short weekend getaway, or choosing a movie night over a walk. These instances show you're balancing fitness with enjoying life. 100% consistency can sometimes be a red flag, suggesting it might be time to ease up and enjoy life's other pleasures.

SEPTEMBER

SUN	MON	TUES	WED	THUR	FRI	SAT
1 ✓	2 ✓	3 ✓	4 ✓	5 ✓	6 ○	7 ✓
8 ✓	9 ✓	10 ✓	11 ○	12 ✓	13 ✓	14 ✓
15 ✓	16 ✓	17 ✓	18 ✓	19 ✓	20 ✓	21 ○
22 ✓	23 ✓	24 ✓	25 ○	26 ✓	27 ✓	28 ✓
29 ✓	30 ✓					

Strength Gains

Not long after graduating from my strength and conditioning degree and moving back to South London from Preston, I developed a strong desire to master the pull-up. My ambitions were clear and became a significant focus of my training:

- Do 3 clean pull-ups with an added 30kg weight strapped to me.
- Do 15 clean bodyweight pull-ups.

These aims shaped that chapter of my training and massively steered my efforts, with both goals being achieved successfully.

Interestingly, until then, I had never considered setting performance goals. The idea of excelling at pull-ups was sudden. What surprised me most was that the aesthetic results I had always pursued were achieved incidentally, but without the usual fixation on looks. This realisation was a lightbulb moment, teaching me a valuable lesson about the benefits of focusing on strength gains.

Nowadays, strength gains hold a special place in my suggestions among the indicators of progress listed. This preference doesn't mean the other progress indicators aren't important, as each can play a crucial role, as I've highlighted. Yet, focusing on strength gains offers a refreshing shift away from aesthetic or weight-focused goals because you're directing your attention to a vital aspect of fitness that deserves attention regardless.

Know that strength improvements, or what you could refer to as "performance goals," allow you to set objectives that, while pushing you towards physical improvements, also gently guide your other goals—like fat loss and improved body composition—into alignment, often without the sometimes exhausting focus that's associated with them–which was exactly what happened to me while training for a better pull-up. Not to mention, it can be enjoyable and motivating when working towards a performance-based goal, too.

Examples of performance goals might include:

- Mastering your first pull-up.
- Completing 10 clean push-ups.
- Deadlifting twice your body weight.
- Squatting half your body weight with a barbell.
- Performing double-figure dumbbell rows.

The beauty of performance goals lies in their adaptability; they can be tailored to fit any strength training experience level, making them a gem in your fitness arsenal.

If you have a specific goal in your workouts, consider setting a performance goal. Determine what you want to achieve, and then figure out your plan and path to success.

Mental Progress

Mental progress is typically the most overlooked aspect of a self-improvement journey because it's less visible than the numbers on the scale or the changes in progress photos.

Here's how mental progress might look:

- You no longer let the scale determine your mood for the day, understanding it's just one piece of data.
- Resisting office treats like pizza, chocolate, or cake becomes less of a struggle, helping you avoid overeating.
- After years of strict dieting, you enjoy occasional ice cream or cookies without feeling guilty.
- Looking at yourself in the mirror or being in photos feels comfortable again.
- You've developed a healthier relationship with exercise, viewing it as a form of self-care rather than a punishment.
- You've learned to appreciate your body's capabilities, focusing on what it can do rather than just how it looks.
- You approach challenges with a problem-solving mindset rather than feeling defeated.
- You celebrate small victories and progress, understanding that consistent, small steps lead to significant long-term results.
- You've cultivated a sense of inner peace and self-acceptance, recognising that your self-worth isn't tied to physical appearance or fitness achievements.

Remember, physical changes without mental growth are usually short-lived. Mental progress is the foundation of lasting change, so it's crucial to celebrate these victories, too!

As we conclude the section on indicators of progress, let's discuss the subject of "Redefining Success",—which could hugely impact whether or not you realise you're moving in the direction you want outside of traditional indicators.

Chapter 14:
Redefining Success

Now, as our time in this coffee shop winds down and our cups hold nothing but coffee stains, let's shift our idea of success.

Think of it like this: similar to how we each have our music genre preferences, success in your fat loss journey is also personal. Of course, wanting to look better aesthetically is great, but it isn't solely about shedding pounds or changing how you look. It's also about the new habits you've formed, the strength you've gained, and the joy of feeling healthier. Success is the many indicators that make this whole experience, not just the endpoint, much like how enjoying our coffee chat isn't just about the drink, but the warmth and connection you and I have shared.

Now, this isn't to say there's anything wrong with wanting to look better naked. I'm all for that if it's what you want. If it gets you to start looking after your health and fitness more, that's amazing. Plus, it's something I fully understand from personal experience. As a teenager, my start in fitness was driven by body dysmorphia and a desire for increased self-confidence.

However, as we mature in our fitness journeys, it becomes apparent that while aesthetic goals have their place, the significance of long-term health, pain-free living, and maintaining functional daily activity hold greater importance.

This realisation marks the transition to viewing health as a journey rather than a mere destination.

Health as a Journey, Not a Destination

While doing a gym induction in Fulham, I'll never forget being asked by Michael, a new gym member who was eager to start strength training, eating well, and being healthier overall: "How long do you think it'll take until I've decided I don't want to make any more progress and maintain what I have?"

It took me aback because his question was the first time I realised that once you start, it forever becomes a journey of continuous self-improvement.

Seeing your health as a journey encourages a shift from an outcome-focused mindset, where immediate goals like losing 10kg as quickly as possible dominate your thoughts and actions. Often, this results in taking drastic and unsustainable measures that, though they might bring short-term results, are detrimental in the long run.

That's why I often suggest that no matter how much you want to change, it can be helpful to think of it as a one-year journey. With this timeline shift in mind, you won't be so obsessed with how quickly you think changes "should" happen. Instead, you'll focus more on the sustainable habits that'll get you there.

Consider the belt system in BJJ as an analogy.

Progressing through the belts—from white to black—signifies growth and improvement, with each belt colour and the stripes earned along the way marking development milestones. However, in BJJ, the focus isn't merely on obtaining the next belt but on consistent practice, learning, and refining skills—the higher belts and stripes are just a byproduct.

This principle applies equally to fitness: rather than fixating on losing a specific amount of weight, the focus should be on consistent actions—such as committing to regular workouts, scheduling walks and following a nutritional plan that works best for you. You'll then find that just like the belts and stripes in BJJ, your fitness goals have a funny way of falling into place, too.

With that cleared up, let's discuss the importance of fat loss being a phase.

Fat Loss is a Phase, Not a Lifestyle

Fat loss is often viewed as a never-ending journey, with many people spending their entire lives pursuing it. However, it's important to recognise that fat loss should be a season—a phase limited to specific periods, whether a few months or a couple of years. It's not something to chase forever.

This idea became clear when I first moved to Japan for 15 months. The disciplined fitness routine I had maintained in South London faced a new challenge when I moved to Tokyo: the countless delicious food options, from the bustling streets of Shibuya to the cosy izakayas of Ikebukuro.

One evening in Shin-Okubo, Tokyo's Korean town, I faced a pivotal choice: stick rigidly to my nutrition plan or embrace the local cuisine with friends and eat more than planned. I decided to enjoy the tasty local dishes, and this choice turned out to be beneficial for my health, marking a shift toward a more balanced approach.

That decision was a turning point. It allowed me to appreciate my time in Japan as a once-in-a-lifetime experience, deserving of a flexible approach to fitness. I continued to exercise and eat nutritious foods but stopped denying myself the joy of Japan's fantastic cuisine. This balance made my time there memorable and reinforced the importance of adjusting your fitness approach to life's circumstances.

This experience is why I've emphasised the need to occasionally shift focus. After several months of consistency, taking a break from relentlessly chasing fat loss can be beneficial for several reasons. It allows your body to recover from a continuous calorie deficit—assuming you've genuinely been cutting calories rather than unintentionally eating more than you realise. Increasing your intake to maintenance or even a slight surplus can provide the energy needed to thrive, boost your daily activity levels, and support real muscle growth.

There are mental benefits, too. The constant mindset of dieting and being in a calorie deficit can be mentally exhausting. Once you've reached your fat loss goals, stepping back—whether temporarily or permanently—can feel liberating.

And it's okay if you gain a little fat during challenging phases. Body fat naturally fluctuates, and that's part of the journey. Some fluctuations in body fat are cyclical. There will be phases where you gain a little more, and then phases when you lose it again—and that's perfectly normal. After our chat, you'll know exactly what to do if you ever want or need to lose body fat again.

Understanding the different seasons of your fitness journey can significantly improve your quality of life, making it more enjoyable and sustainable in the long term.

Now, let's move on to the final part of our chat before wrapping things up.

The Ripple Effect of Healthy Habits

Have you heard the story of the infamous Colombian drug lord Pablo Escobar and his hippos?

For context, Pablo was fascinated with exotic animals, including 4 hippos—one male and 3 females—that he illegally imported to his private estate. After his death, these hippos escaped into the wild. Without any natural predators in Colombia, they thrived in their new environment, multiplying far beyond their original numbers, leading to massive unforeseen ecological impacts on the local habitat.

This story sets the stage for understanding how seemingly minor changes can have massive ripple effects—much like the choices you'll make in your fat loss journey. Adopting a healthy habit can ignite an enormous chain reaction, leading to broader positive changes and improving overall quality of life.

Remember the cycle of "Action → Results → Motivation" that we mentioned earlier?

The ripple effect is similar, where taking an initial step can lead to unexpected and motivating outcomes.

For instance, imagine you start tracking your calories out of curiosity and realise your usual breakfast and lunch are each heavy 1,200-calorie meals. You then decide to adjust your diet to include more nutrient-dense, lower-calorie foods and leaner protein. After maintaining these changes for 3 weeks, you notice a significant drop in weight, which motivates you to utilise your gym membership for strength training 3 times a week. This new routine not only helps in fat loss but also alleviates the chronic lower back pain you've experienced, making daily activities and time with your kids

171

much easier. Your improved activity levels increase your presence in their lives, creating cherished memories.

All these positive changes started from the simple decision to track your calories for a few days.

These ripple effect examples remind us of the potential impact of small beginnings on life-changing outcomes. Sometimes, the best starting point involves modest adjustments rather than drastic changes, which can be overwhelming and lead to quitting.

I've always said that if you regularly tell yourself you'll start your fitness journey "next Monday," it's a sign that the changes you typically try to implement are too drastic. Starting with smaller, more manageable habits could be the answer here.

Concluding our discussion, I'll share some final thoughts.

Chapter 15:
Concluding Thoughts

As we find ourselves with empty coffee cups that have been untouched for a while, and with the coffee shop nearing its closing time, it's time to share my final thoughts so we can wrap up and head home.

I urge you not to let our chat become "just another piece of advice in your collection." The strategies, discussions, and tips we've covered only work if you put them into practice. There's a kind of paralysis that comes from constantly gathering knowledge without ever implementing it. Don't let that happen—take what we've discussed and start applying it today.

You don't need another course, podcast, book, video, or seminar. What you need now is to put what you've learned into motion. After all, the effectiveness of any plan comes down to consistent action.

You already know what you need to do. I'm rooting for you.

If you enjoyed this read and want to inquire about becoming a 1-2-1 online fitness member to work alongside me, head here: kairos.online/inquiry-form

Alternatively, if you'd simply like to stay in touch, go here to sign up for my weekly emails: kairos.online/newsletter

I usually send emails once or twice a week—though on a particularly exciting week, it might be three—with tips on nutrition, fitness, training, motivation, and more. And every once in a while, I'll probably try to sell you something—but that's only because I genuinely believe what I offer can change your life, and I'd be doing you a disservice by not having you on board.

Helpful Links

kairos.online/inquiry-form - The inquiry form for working with me and becoming a 1-2-1 online fitness member

kairos.online/calorie-calculator - My free calorie calculator

kairos.online/pdf-guides - The free workout plan and other free fitness guides

kairos.online/newsletter - Sign-up for my email list

Acknowledgements Page

A big thank you to my family, including my amazing grandparents, lovely parents, wonderful wife, amazing sister, fantastic brother, awesome godson, tremendous aunts and uncles, and all my other relatives. There are far too many to name—over 100!—but please know you're all appreciated.

A heartfelt thank you to my closest friends. I genuinely cherish the friendships I have with each of you.

Thanks to Madalena Rodrigues, Kathleen Ann Staniford, and Amy Keane for changing the trajectory of my life during a pivotal moment in my teenage years. I was lost.

A special thank you to Susan Niebergall for her generous guidance on publishing a first book and to Jordan Syatt and Mike Vacanti for being such great business and coaching mentors.

A huge thank you to Bob Hoover, Marcus Balogun, José Catanho, Lucas Peres-Johnson, Shola Adedo, and Ed Rushworth for proofreading and offering suggestions on individual chapters. Bob, in particular, also brought a coach's perspective to the process, which I truly appreciate.

My gratitude also goes to Myles Asiedu-Nesbeth and Miguel Mendes for their insights and suggestions on various chapters from a fellow coach's perspective, and to Akim Montrose-Francis and Tiffany Shand for proofreading the entire book—which I know was no small feat.

About Leo, the Author

I was born and raised in South London, England, but my parents are from Lisbon, Portugal. Although South London is ultimately home, I have also lived in Preston, Burlington (V.T.), Tokyo, Osaka, the Alentejo region of Portugal, and Lisbon. Each location offered unique experiences, shaping who I am and what I share with you today.

My fitness journey began when I was kicked out of sixth form at 17. At that time, I wasn't in a great place mentally. I felt insecure about my appearance due to a compounding of inactivity, lack of nutrition awareness, feeling physically heavy, and having low confidence. Because of this, I started attending a gym to lose weight and gain muscle. Although it took a long time to figure out how to approach my training and nutrition correctly, I enjoyed the process.

As I delved deeper into training, research, certifications, and internships, friends, family, and even strangers began asking me questions. That's when I realised I loved helping others—people like you—get stronger, lose fat, and achieve their fitness goals. With so much misinformation out there, I felt compelled to help. So, I became a personal trainer, and the rest is history.

I hold a master's degree in Strength and Conditioning from the University of Central Lancashire in Preston, England, and I've studied nutrition in-depth during my study abroad at the University of Vermont, USA, where I took several courses that helped me understand how nutrition impacts everyday health and fitness. I've also completed internships with professional football clubs like Fulham FC and Preston North End FC, and worked with the Wigan Warriors rugby team—but what truly drives me is helping people improve their lives through fitness.

Over the years, I've coached both in-person at gyms like Nuffield Health and online, working with clients from all walks of life. My goal has always been to help people fit health into their busy lives—whether that means finding time to exercise, making smarter food choices, or simply feeling more confident in their own skin.

Outside of fitness, sushi and fried chicken are my favourite foods, and it's not even close. I study Japanese using textbooks, phone apps, podcasts, watching videos and conversations with friends. Brazilian Jiu-Jitsu is another hobby I enjoy. Though inconsistently, I enjoy a game of chess. Nowadays, you can find me near Lisbon enjoying espressos, reading my Kindle and working alongside my 1-2-1 online fitness members.

Milton Keynes UK
Ingram Content Group UK Ltd.
UKHW022021261024
450212UK00010B/99

9 789893 591314